The Ultimate Ulcerative Colitis Cookbook

Recipes To Cure Ulcerative Colitis and Reduce Inflammation!

By: Logan King

Copyright © 2021 by Logan King

Edition Notice

The author has taken any step to make sure this book is accurate and safe. Every info is checked. However, every step you take following the book do it with caution and on your own accord.

If you end up with a copied and illegal version of this book please delete it and get the original. This will support the author to create even better books for everyone. Also, if possible report where you have found the illegal version.

This book is under copyright license which means no one is allowed to make any changes, prints, copies, republish or sell it except for the author.

Table of Contents

Introduction 7

What is the Anti-inflammatory Diet for Ulcerative Colitis? 10

How Does the Anti-Inflammatory Diet Work? 12

What Foods Should You Avoid on the Anti-Inflammatory Diet? 13

Foods to Enjoy on the Anti-Inflammatory Diet 14

Benefits of The Anti-Inflammatory Diet 16

Breakfast 17

    1. Fruity Flaxseed Breakfast Bowl 18

    2. Cinnamon & Coco Milk Muffins with Specially Prepared Sweet Potato 20

    3. Pumpkin Puree Porridge 23

    4. Choco Chia Banana Bowl 25

    5. Sweet and Savory Breakfast Hash 28

    6. Healthy Chickpea Scramble Stuffed Sweet Potatoes 31

    7. Green Smoothie Bowl 34

    8. Fruity Bowl 36

    9. Golden-Orange Overnight Oats 38

10. Banana & Peanut Butter Smoothie 40

11. Egg & Sweet Potato Breakfast Hash 42

12. Apple & Banana Pancakes 45

Mains 48

13. Curried Chicken 'n Rice 49

14. Rice Noodles & Tofu 52

15. Chicken & Cheese Pasta Salad 55

16. Tasty Salmon Burger 58

17. Roast Tarragon Chicken 60

18. Niçoise Lettuce-Free "Salad" 63

19. Spaghetti Squash Boats 65

20. Chicken Piccata on Pasta 69

21. Turkey with Thyme & Sage Sausage 72

22. Blackened Chicken Breast 74

23. Creamy Pesto Chicken 77

24. Salmon and Dill Pâté 80

25. Vegetable and Chicken Stir Fry 82

26. Curried Shrimp and Vegetables 84

27. Mango Chicken Meal 86

28. Mediterranean Tuna-Spinach Salad 88

29. Lemony Mussels 90

Snacks and Appetizer 92

30. Green Bean Snack 93

31. Avocado and Pepper Hummus 95

32. Easy Eggplant Spread 97

33. Creamy Artichoke Spread 99

34. Balsamic Onion Snack 101

35. Sweet Paprika Oysters 103

36. Citrus Oyster Platter 105

37. Salmon and Avocado Wraps 107

38. Radish Chips 109

39. Avocado Cream 111

Desserts 113

40. Orange Sorbet 114

41. Lemon Cake with Pecans 116

42. Pineapple and Orange Smoothie 118

43. Coconut Ice Cream 120

Conclusion 122

About the Author 124

Appendices 125

Introduction

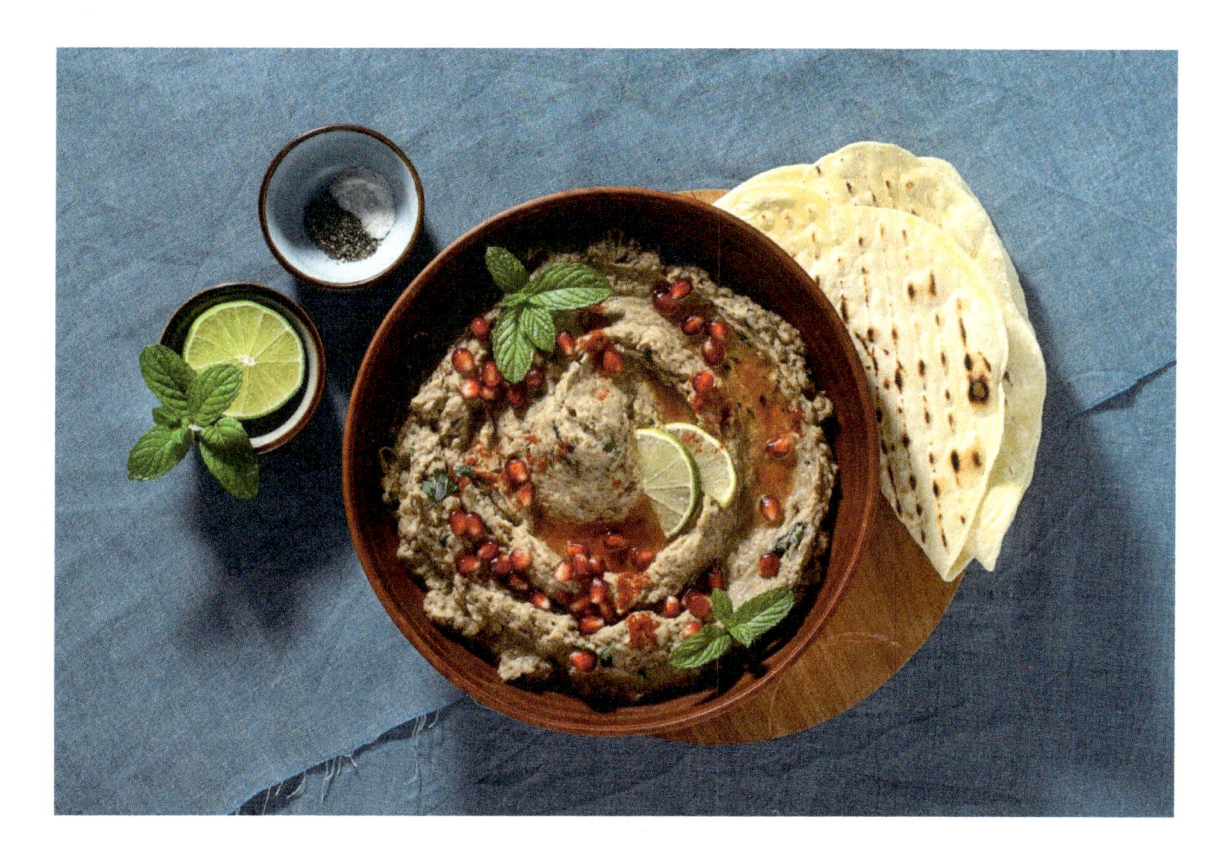

Ulcerative colitis is a chronic disease of the large intestine that causes continual ulcers, or open sores, in the colon. Ulcerative colitis can be a debilitating and sometimes life-threatening condition. It's estimated that 1 million Americans suffer from ulcerative colitis (UC). UC often begins as an intermittent illness lasting weeks or months, followed by periods without symptoms. More than half of those afflicted with UC have mild symptoms but need medical care for severe attacks.

To most effectively manage this illness, proper education is essential. UC patients need to learn about their disease, how to manage it, and what preventive measures they can take to avoid painful flare-ups. The more you know about your illness, the better equipped you are to help your doctor make decisions about your care.

The benefits of living a healthy lifestyle, including a well-balanced diet and regular exercise, will help with disease management and recovery while reducing symptoms and reducing dependency on medications.

There are two types of ulcerative colitis:

1) Crohn's Disease: This is much more common than UC (60-80% compared to 20-30%). It usually causes abdominal pain, rectal bleeding, diarrhea, and weight loss which is sometimes severe but rarely leads to death. It can occur at any age but seems to affect young people.

2) UC: This is more common in elderly people and is somewhat non-specific (24% of patients). Symptoms are often milder.

Other types of inflammatory bowel disease can also exist, such as ulcerative proctitis, granulomatous colitis, and collagenous colitis. These are less common than UC&Crohn's disease and usually cause fewer symptoms or no symptoms at all. They may be accompanied by a skin disorder called Behçet's syndrome.

Some symptoms of Crohn's disease are similar to those of UC. Therefore, a doctor may mistake them for one another if you also have symptoms of the other type (UC), such as abdominal cramping, diarrhea, weight loss, and rectal bleeding.

While the two types of inflammatory bowel disease (Crohn's disease and UC) have many similarities, there are also important differences between them.

1) UC is usually confined to the colon, whereas Crohn's disease can affect other parts of the digestive tract.

2) The cause of Crohn's disease is not known, but both types may result from genetically determined changes in immune function and/or environmental factors such as smoking or infections with certain viruses or bacteria that damage tissue.

3) While both types of inflammatory bowel disease may cause diarrhea, Crohn's disease tends to produce more bloody stools and is more likely to cause abdominal pain than UC.

4) Small intestine involvement in UC is much more common than in Crohn's disease (majority of patients have small intestine involvement)

5) Ulcerative colitis typically causes fewer complications that are often related to the severity of the condition or the patient's age compared with Crohn's disease, where serious complications can occur at any age.

6) The clinical course of ulcerative colitis may be faster than in Crohn's disease as it does not usually stay present for long periods before treatment starts.

Also, UC is an inflammatory bowel disease that specifically affects the colon. It can only affect the large intestine and not other parts of the gastrointestinal tract, such as the small intestine and stomach. The inflammatory response caused by UC involves all layers of the intestinal wall.

What is the Anti-inflammatory Diet for Ulcerative Colitis?

Ulcerative colitis is a type of inflammatory bowel disease (IBD) which means that the colon and large intestine become inflamed or irritated. This leads to ulcers, bleeding, and ulcerative colitis may even cause rectal bleeding. This condition can be extremely painful, and many people are unable to work or maintain a social life because of it. The anti-inflammatory diet for ileocolonic Crohn's disease is an important part of managing this condition. Those with ileocolonic Crohn's must avoid foods rich in xanthine compounds like coffee, tea, chocolate, tomato sauce, garlic, and pyruvic acid found in vegetables, including cabbage, broccoli, and broccoli cauliflower, and Brussels sprouts.

According to the National Institutes of Health, inflammatory bowel disease is when the digestive tract becomes swollen and inflamed. Crohn's disease may also cause ulcerations, fistulas, fissures, or abscesses in the lining of the intestines. It causes abdominal pain, diarrhea, and fecal incontinence; it can also cause a loss of appetite, fever, and weight loss. Ulcerative colitis is another form of inflammatory bowel disease, but it only affects the colon and rectum. It causes inflammation as well as sores and open wounds, which will eventually scar if left untreated.

There is no cure for inflammatory bowel disease, but there are treatments that can help prevent flare-ups. The anti-inflammatory diet is one of these treatments, and it can also help to decrease diarrhea, cramping, abdominal pain, and bleeding. There are other foods that the anti-inflammatory diet for ileocolonic Crohn's disease calls for, including probiotics, fruits, nuts (almonds, walnuts, or pistachio), seeds (flax, chia, or hemp), fish, and high-quality protein such as organic chicken or turkey.

There are many health risks associated with inflammatory bowel disease; in fact, some believe that it lowers life expectancy. The anti-inflammatory diet helps to prevent symptoms of Crohn's disease, but it is also very beneficial when used in conjunction with other treatments. Some may choose to avoid certain foods, but this should be done under the advice of a doctor. If you are following the anti-inflammatory diet, then you will need to rely on food that is high in fiber, low in fat, and rich in fruit and vegetables such as green leafy vegetables, whole grains, fruits, olive oil, and protein such as organic chicken or turkey.

How Does the Anti-Inflammatory Diet Work?

The anti-inflammatory diet reduces intestinal inflammation by restricting foods that increase the levels of harmful chemicals in the body. This is done by reducing the potential production and side effects of inflammatory chemicals like histamine, leukotrienes, and prostaglandins. The anti-inflammatory diet for ileocolonic Crohn's disease also helps to prevent outbreaks of intestinal inflammation by reducing the rate at which food gets absorbed into the blood supply, where it can begin to cause damage. This means that the anti-inflammatory diet will reduce the number of harmful chemicals that enter the body. The diet also reduces inflammation by reducing levels of bacterial toxins like LPS found in some food products. LPS can cause inflammation and a wide range of symptoms, including abdominal pain, diarrhea, and fecal incontinence.

The anti-inflammatory diet is one of many recommended treatments for Crohn's disease. Patients should speak to their doctor about any other dietary changes that they would like to make while they are following it, such as increasing fiber intake, getting more exercise, or using medication to help lessen inflammation.

What Foods Should You Avoid on the Anti-Inflammatory Diet?

The anti-inflammatory diet is very specific about what foods you can eat and what you should avoid. It is important to understand the specifics of this diet so that you do not get confused when shopping or eating out. The following foods must be avoided: high-fat dairy products such as cream, butter, cheese, and full-fat ice cream, as well as red meat, sugar, and processed wheat products. The following foods are permitted: fish such as salmon, egg whites, low-fat yogurt (plain), and plain popcorn.

Foods to Enjoy on the Anti-Inflammatory Diet

Fish. This includes salmon, tuna, sardines, and other coldwater fish. You should aim for at least two small servings of fish per week.

Nuts and seeds. This includes walnuts, almonds, sunflower seeds, pumpkin seeds, and chia seeds. It is recommended that you eat a handful a day to help with inflammation.

Omega-3 pills. Most people do not get enough omega 3 in their diet without the help of supplements. These pills are usually made from fish oil, or flaxseed oil can help with inflammation and other symptoms as well, such as pain management.

Probiotics. These are living microorganisms that help to keep your gut healthy. The most common probiotics used by Crohn's patients are the Lactobacillus and Bifidobacterium species. They can help to prevent inflammation in your intestines as well as reduce the risk of diarrhea and abdominal pain.

Prebiotics. These are fiber-rich foods that are designed to help the intestines stay healthy. Foods like onions, garlic, leeks, and sweet potatoes should be included in your diet.

White potatoes and starchy vegetables such as winter squashes. These are both starchier versions of white potato, but they do not cause inflammation, so they can be eaten without restriction on the anti-inflammatory diet for ileocolonic Crohn's disease. You can include other starchy vegetables in your diets, such as yams and taro.

Gluten-free whole grain products. These are the best options to eat on this plan, particularly for patients who need to cut down on the gluten content of their diets due to celiac disease or gluten sensitivity.

Benefits of The Anti-Inflammatory Diet

Perhaps the main benefits of using this type of diet are the following:

- Reduces inflammation, which leads to a significant improvement in health. Reduces symptoms of ulcerative colitis.
- Reduces uncomfortable side effects associated with treatment with corticosteroids.
- Reduces the risk of getting colorectal cancer (the second most frequent cause of death in males).
- Reduces the risk of developing diabetes, cardiovascular disease, and cataracts.
- It also delays aging and improves immunity.

Breakfast

1. Fruity Flaxseed Breakfast Bowl

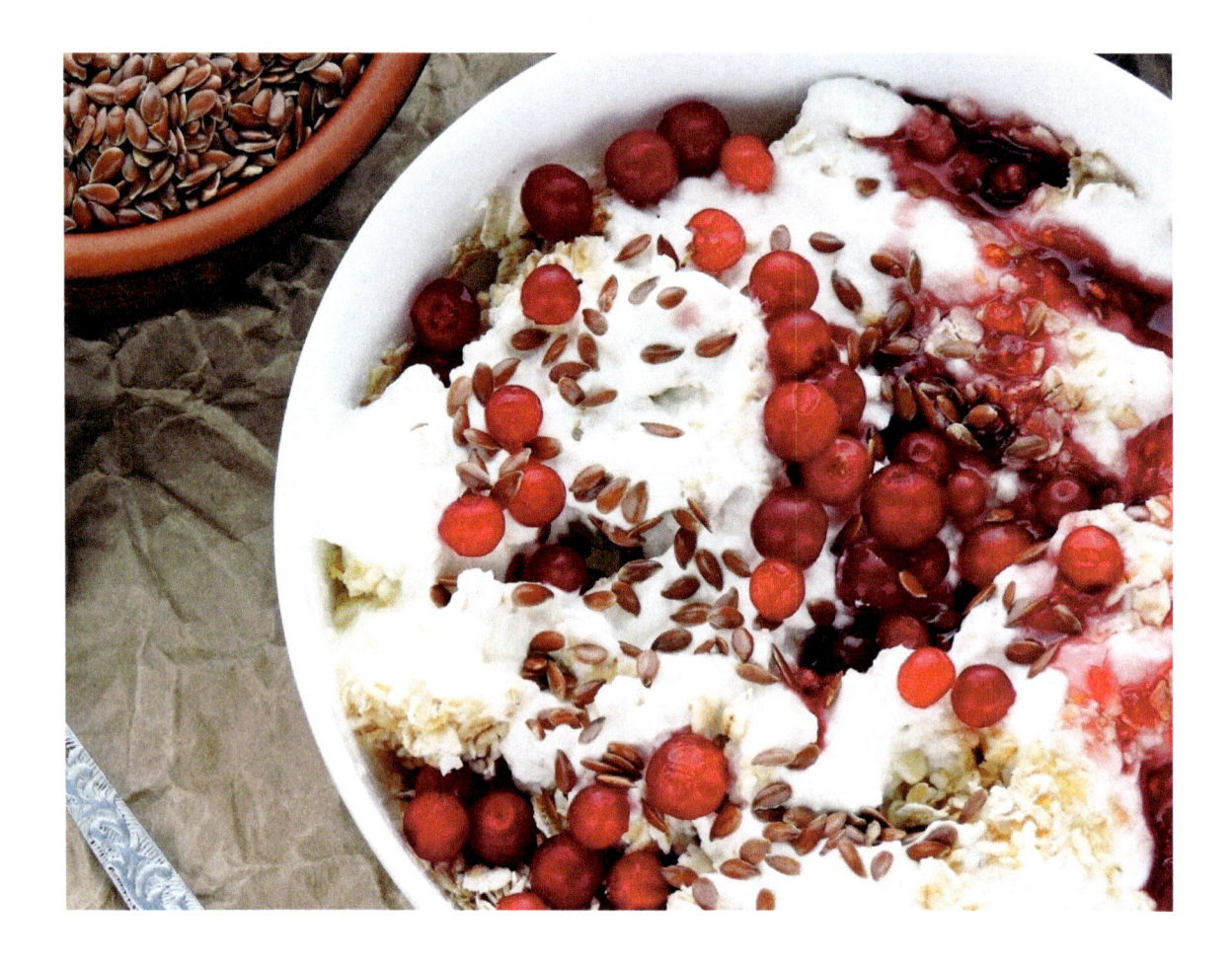

Fruity Flaxseed Breakfast Bowl is a blend of gluten-free and vegan ingredients that make for an excellent breakfast.

Preparation Time: 8-minutes

Cooking Time: 5-minutes

Servings: 1

Ingredients:

For the Porridge:

- ¼-cup flaxseeds, freshly ground
- ¼-tsp cinnamon, ground
- 1-cup almond or coconut milk
- 1-pc medium banana, mashed
- A pinch of fine-grained sea salt

For the Toppings:

- Blueberries, fresh or defrosted
- Walnuts, chopped raw
- Pure maple syrup (optional)

Directions:

In a medium-sized saucepan placed over medium heat, combine all the porridge ingredients. Stir constantly for 5 minutes or until the porridge thickens and comes to a low boil.

Transfer the cooked porridge to a serving bowl. Garnish with the toppings and pour a bit of maple syrup if you want it a little sweeter.

Nutrition: Calories: 780 Fat: 26g Protein: 39g Sodium: 270mg Total Carbs: 117.5g Dietary Fiber: 20g Net Carbs: 97.5g

2. Cinnamon & Coco Milk Muffins with Specially Prepared Sweet Potato

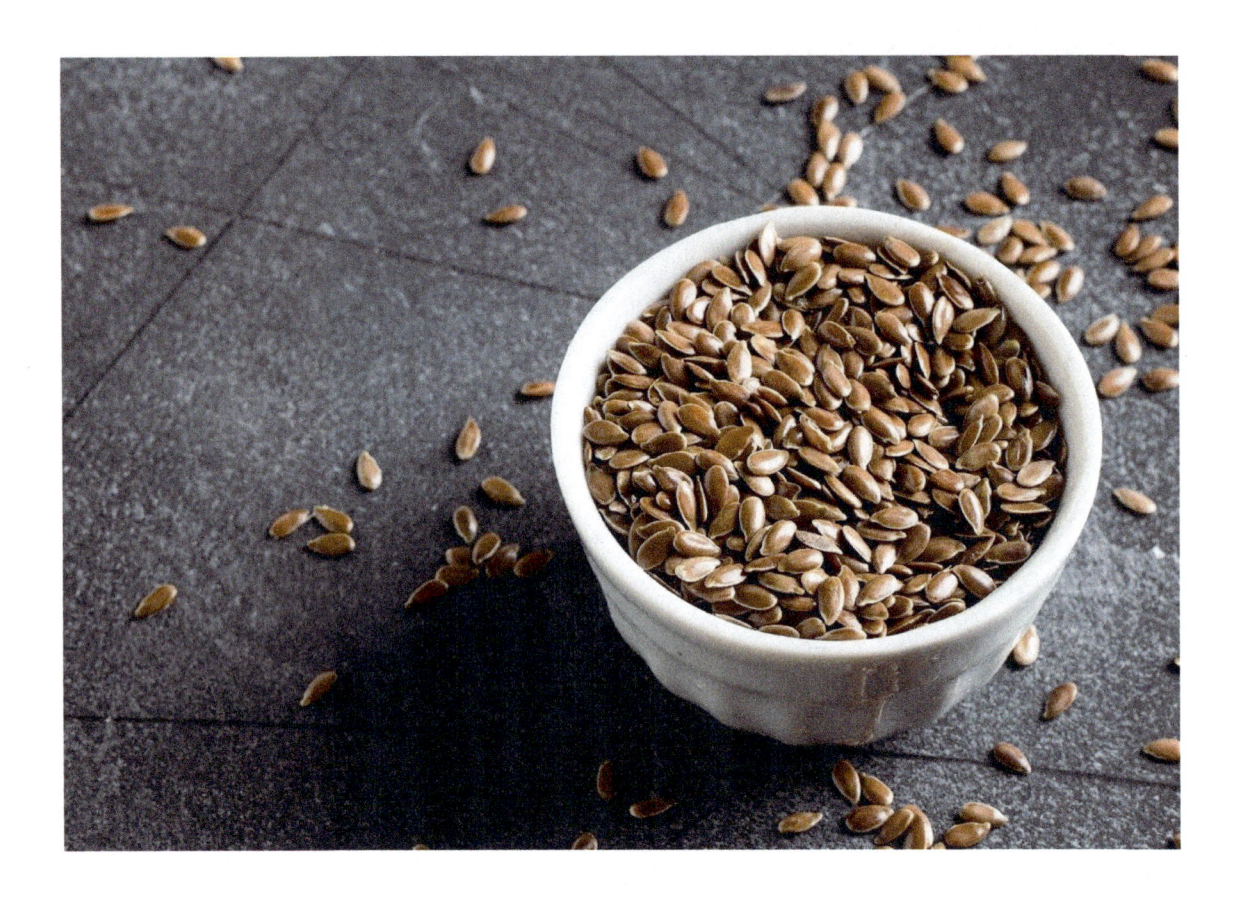

This is a light, moist, and delicious gluten-free muffin recipe that can be enjoyed as a breakfast or an anytime snack.

Preparation Time: 25-minutes

Cooking Time: 35-minutes

Servings: 4

Ingredients:

- Coconut oil for greasing
- 1-pc small sweet potato, roasted
- 3-tbsp flaxseed, ground, soaked in ½-cup water
- 2-tbsp olive oil
- ¾-cup coconut milk
- ½-cup pure maple syrup
- 1/8-tsp cloves, ground
- 1/8-tsp nutmeg, ground
- ¼-cup coconut flour
- ½-tsp Himalayan salt
- 1-cup brown rice flour
- 1-tbsp baking powder
- 1-tbsp cinnamon, ground
- 1-tsp ginger, ground
- 1-tsp turmeric, ground

Directions:

Preheat your oven to 400°F. Meanwhile, grease your muffin tray lightly with coconut oil.

By using a wooden skewer, pierce about a dozen holes around the sweet potato. Cook it for an hour or until soft.

Slice the potato crosswise and scoop out its flesh into a large mixing bowl. Pour the soaked flaxseed—combining the specially prepared egg mixed with the potato—olive oil, coconut milk, and maple syrup. Mix well to a smooth consistency.

Stir in all of the dry ingredients in another mixing bowl. Mix well until thoroughly combined. Blend the dry and wet mixtures, and mix well until fully incorporated.

Fill each section of the muffin tray up to 2/3 full. Put the tray on the oven's middle rack. Bake for 35 minutes or until the muffins turn golden brown.

Tips/Notes:

You can replace ground flaxseeds with ground chia seeds. You can also substitute raw or unpasteurized honey for maple syrup.

When preparing the meal ahead, you can freeze the muffins and serve them whenever or as you please.

Nutrition: Calories: 510 Fat: 17g Protein: 25.5g Sodium: 320mg Total Carbs: 73.4g Dietary Fiber: 9.7g Net Carbs: 63.7g

3. Pumpkin Puree Porridge

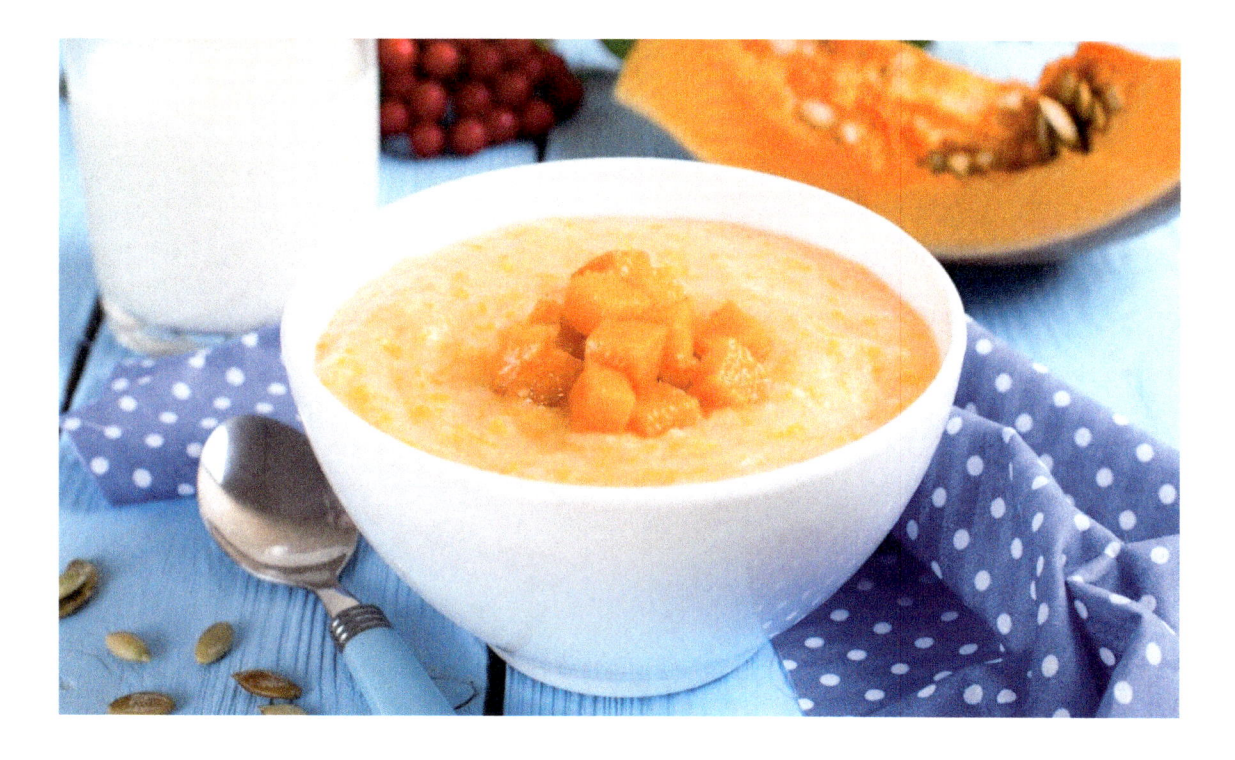

Pumpkin Puree Porridge Recipe is a delicious porridge that takes pumpkin puree and spices to make an easy and healthy single-serving breakfast. It's perfect for fall or as a quick weeknight meal.

Preparation Time: 1-minute

Cooking Time: 20-minutes

Servings: 1

Ingredients:

- 1-cup water
- 1/3-cup rolled oats
- 1-tbsp chia seeds
- 1-tbsp cocoa powder, unsweetened
- ½-tsp cinnamon
- ½-pc banana, ripe, sliced
- ¼-cup pumpkin puree
- ¼-tsp vanilla extract
- ¼-cup egg whites

Directions:

In a small pot, pour a cup of water, and bring it to a boil. Upon boiling, add in the oats, chia seeds, cocoa powder, and cinnamon. Stir well until thoroughly combined. Cover the pot. Bring to a simmer for a minute.

Add in the banana, and cook further for 5 minutes. Stir periodically to break up the banana slices. As soon as the mixture absorbs about a quarter of the water, pour in the pumpkin puree. Stir the mixture slowly, and cook further for a couple of minutes.

As the mixture absorbs the water almost entirely, add the vanilla and egg whites. Whisk for about 3 minutes until thoroughly combined. Return the lid to the pot and cook for 5 minutes more.

Serve hot with your choice of toppings.

Nutrition: Calories: 197 Fat: 6.5g Protein: 9.8g Sodium: 10mg Total Carbs: 33g Dietary Fiber: 8.4g Net Carbs: 24.6g

4. Choco Chia Banana Bowl

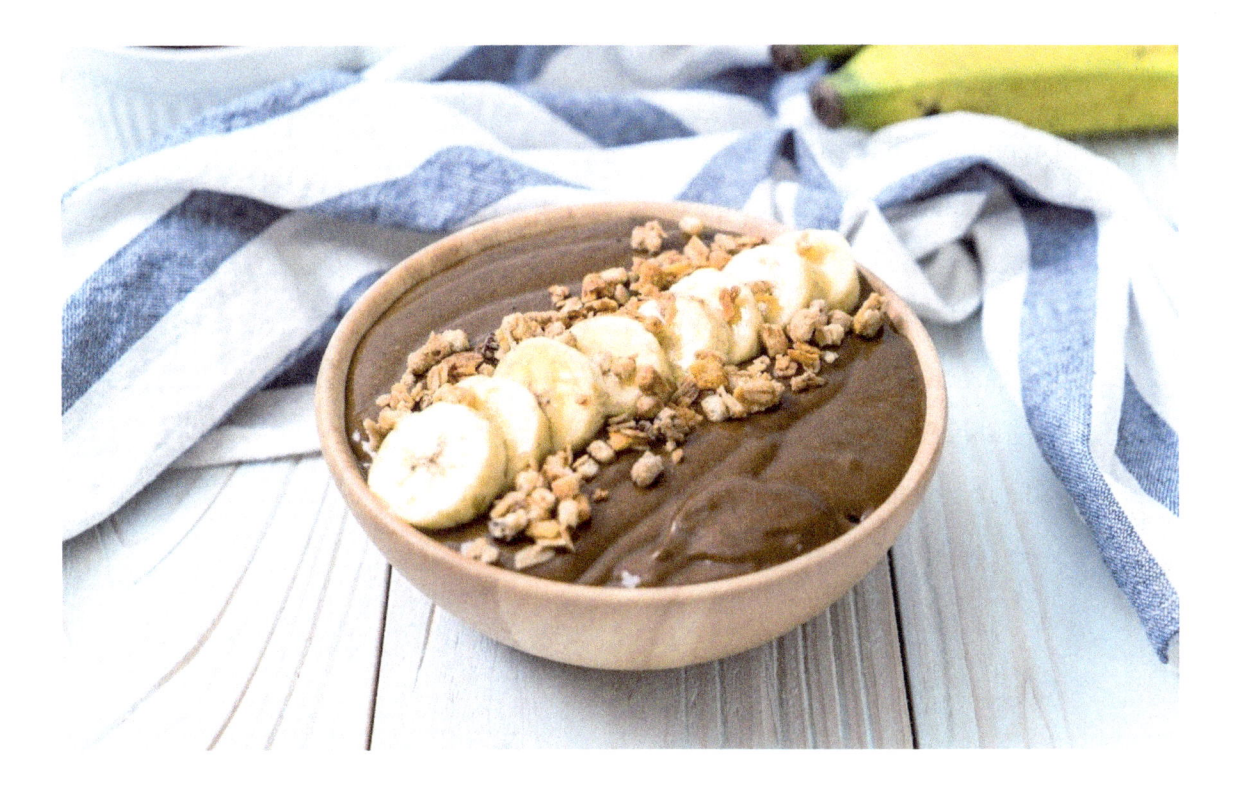

Chocolate Chia Banana Bowl is a vegan, gluten-free, and super healthy dessert recipe that you can whip up in less than 40 minutes. It is also easy and requires only a few ingredients.

Preparation Time: 30 minutes

Cooking Time: 0-minutes

Servings: 3

Ingredients:

- ½-cup chia seeds
- 1-pc large banana, very ripe
- ½-tsp pure vanilla extract
- 2-cups almond milk, unsweetened
- 1-tbsp cacao powder
- 2-tbsp raw honey or maple syrup
- 2-tbsp cacao nibs for mixing in
- 2-tbsps chocolate chips for mixing in
- 1-pc large banana, sliced for mixing in

Directions:

Combine the chia seeds and banana in a mixing bowl. By using a fork, mash the banana and mix well until thoroughly combined. Pour in the vanilla and almond milk. Whisk until no more lumps appear.

Pour half of the mix into a glass container, and cover it. Add the cacao and syrup to the remaining half mixture in the bowl. Mix well until fully incorporated. Pour this mixture into another glass container, and cover it. Refrigerate overnight in both containers or for at least 4 hours.

To serve, layer the chilled chia puddings equally in three serving bowls. Alternate the layers with the ingredients for mixing-in.

Tips/Notes:

You can store the chia puddings or the assembled meal in your refrigerator for up to 5 days.

Nutrition: Calories: 293 Fat: 9.7g Protein: 14.6g Sodium: 35mg Total Carbs: 43.1g Dietary Fiber: 6.5g Net Carbs: 36.6g

5. Sweet and Savory Breakfast Hash

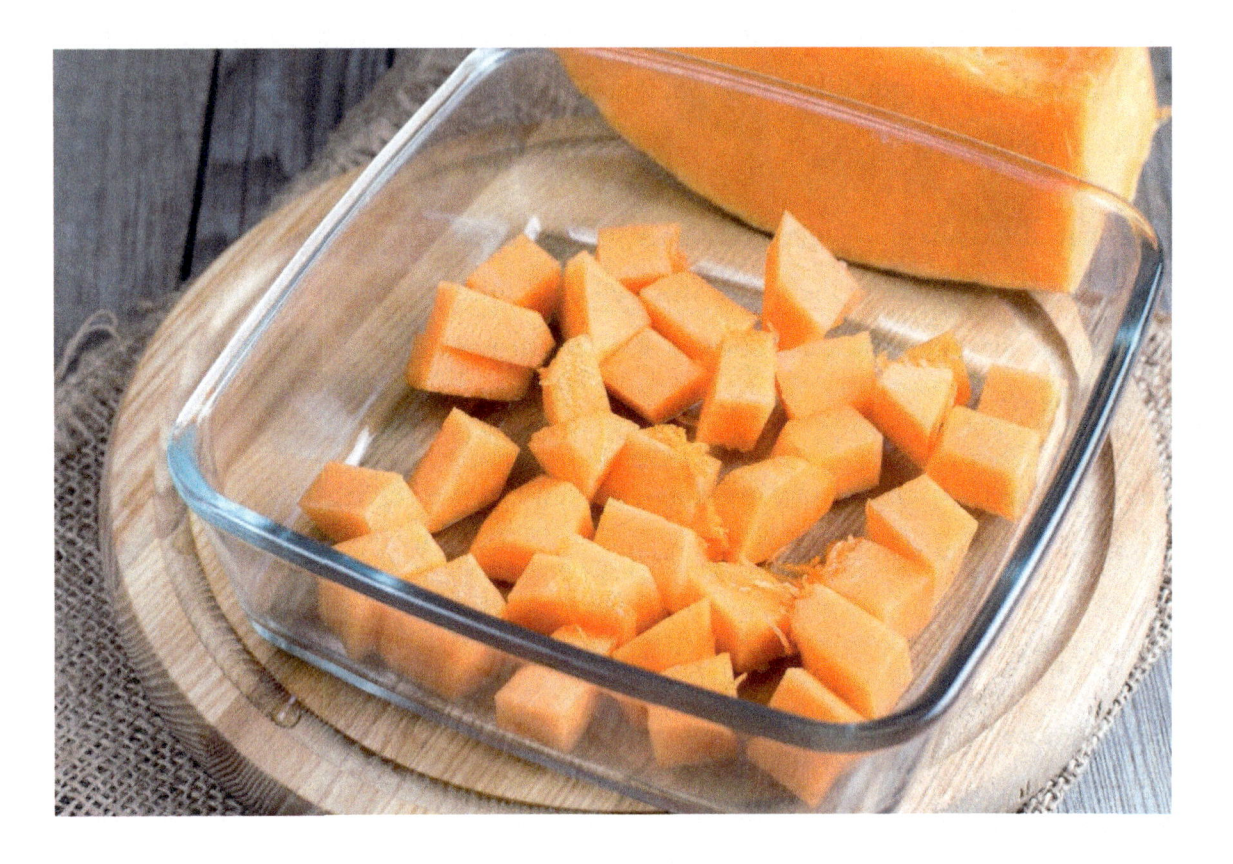

If you have never heard of this recipe before, it is a good recipe for breakfast. This is a savory and sweet breakfast idea that takes very little time to make. It is great for those who are looking for something quick and easy in the morning.

Preparation Time: 10 minutes

Cooking Time: 15 minutes

Servings: 2

Ingredients:

Ingredients for the turkey:

- ¼ tsp cinnamon
- ¼ tsp thyme (dried)
- ½ tbsp coconut oil
- ½ lb. ground turkey
- Sea salt

Ingredients for the hash:

- ¼ tsp garlic powder
- ¼ tsp thyme (dried)
- ¼ tsp turmeric
- 1/3 tsp ginger (powdered)
- ½ tsp cinnamon
- ½ tbsp coconut oil
- ¼ cup of carrots (shredded)
- 1 cup of butternut squash (cubed, you can also use sweet potato)
- 1 cup of spinach (you can also use other types of greens)
- ½ onion (chopped)
- 1 small apple (peeled, cored, chopped)
- 1 small zucchini (chopped)
- Sea salt

Directions:

In a skillet, warm half of the coconut oil over medium-high heat.

Add the turkey and cook until it's browned.

While cooking, season the meat with the spices and mix well.

Once cooked, move the turkey onto a plate.

Add the remaining coconut oil into the skillet, along with the onion.

Sauté the onion until softened for about 2 to 3 minutes.

Add the apple, carrots, squash, and zucchini and cook until softened for about 4 to 5 minutes.

Add the spinach and continue cooking until the leaves wilt.

Add the cooked turkey, along with the hash seasonings, then continue mixing. Taste the hash and adjust the seasonings according to your taste.

Spoon the hash onto serving plates and serve immediately.

Nutrition: Calories: 1284 Fat: 103.02g Protein: 62.02g Sodium: 184mg Total Carbs: 28.23g

6. Healthy Chickpea Scramble Stuffed Sweet Potatoes

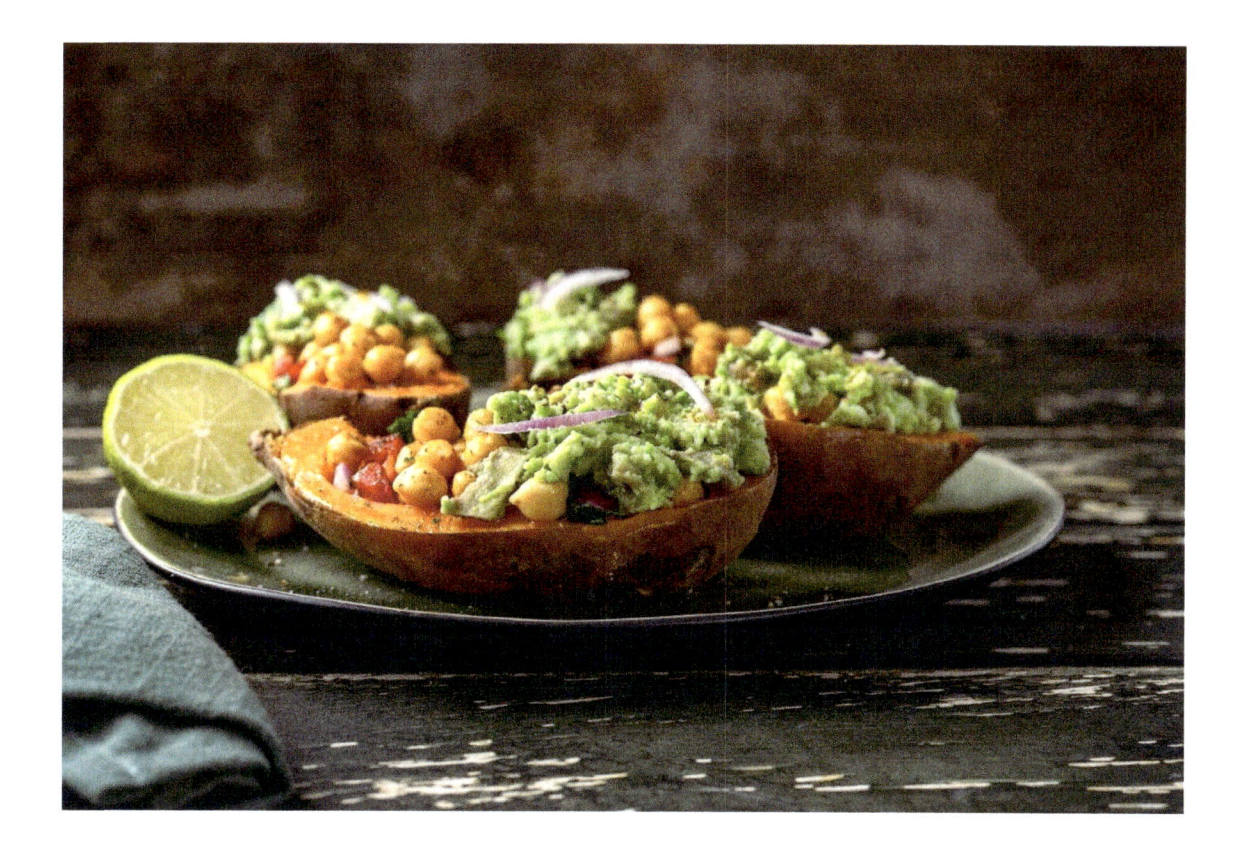

A healthy, protein-rich, vegan alternative to scrambled eggs. This dish can be made with tofu or chickpeas. Do not worry if you are not a fan of sweet potatoes. This dish can also be served on toast or over rice.

Preparation Time: 5 minutes

Cooking Time: 20 minutes

Servings: 2

Ingredients:

Ingredients for the scramble:

- ½ tsp avocado oil
- ½ tsp turmeric
- 1 cup of chickpeas (soaked overnight, boiled for an hour, drained, and dried; you can also use canned, but you must first rinse, drain, and dry)
- ¼ small onion (diced)
- 2 cloves of garlic (minced)
- Sea salt

Ingredients for the kale:

- ½ tsp avocado oil
- ½ tsp garlic (minced)
- 1 cup of kale leaves (stems removed, cut into small pieces)
- Ingredients for assembling:
- ½ avocado (sliced)
- 2 small sweet potatoes (baked)

Directions:

In a pan, add the avocado oil over medium heat, along with the garlic and onions.

Cook for about 3 to 4 minutes until softened.

Add the chickpeas, turmeric, and salt, then continue cooking for about 10 more minutes. To avoid drying the mixture out, you may add teaspoons of water.

Mash about 2/3 of the chickpeas using a wooden spoon to make a scrambled texture.

Take the pan off the heat and set it aside.

In a separate pan, add the avocado oil over medium heat, along with the garlic and kale.

Cook for about 5 minutes, until soft, then take the pan off the heat.

Slice one baked sweet potato in half and use a spoon to scoop out the center.

Spoon half of the chickpea scramble into the baked sweet potato and top with half of the softened kale.

Top with half of the avocado slices.

Repeat the assembling steps for the other baked sweet potato.

Serve immediately and enjoy.

Nutrition: Calories: 275 Fat: 11.76g Protein: 8.31g Sodium: 190mg Total Carbs: 37.34g

7. Green Smoothie Bowl

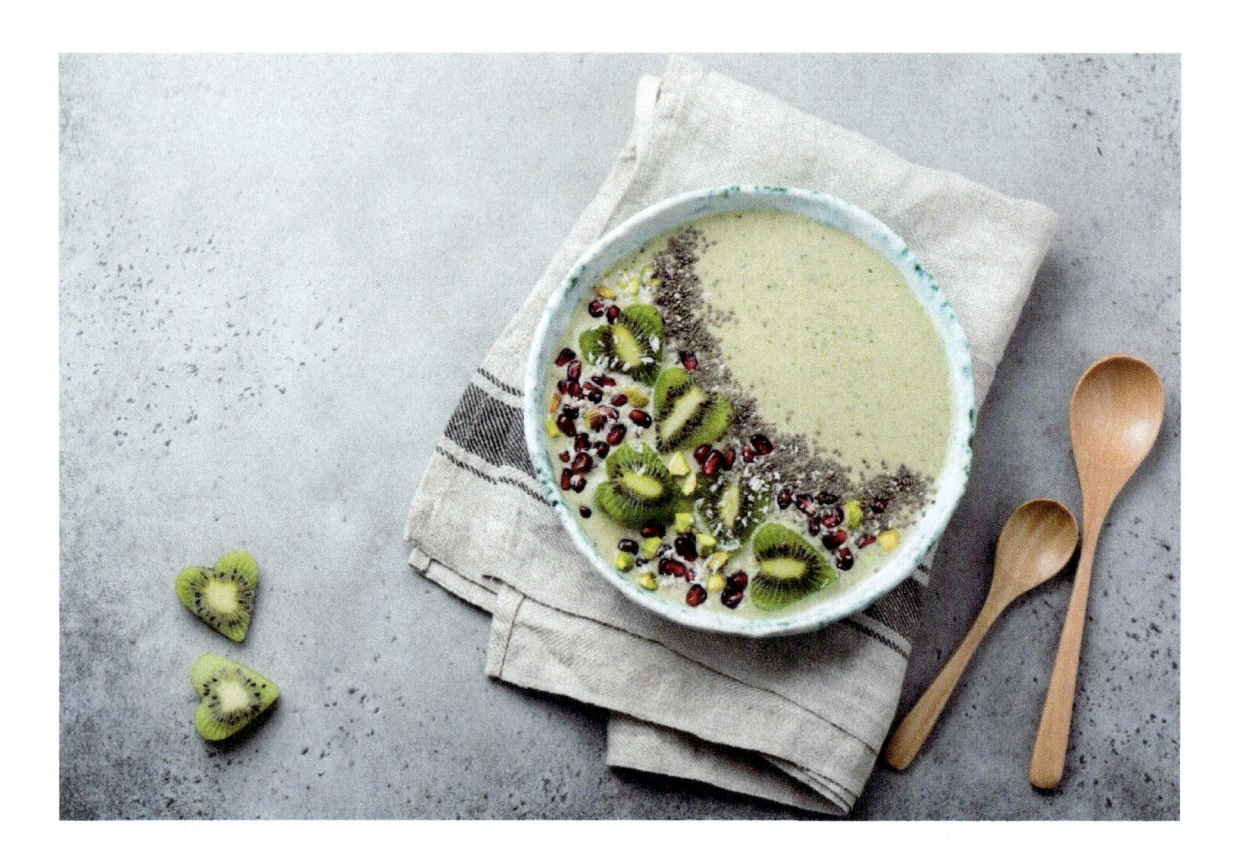

This is a recipe for a green smoothie bowl. It's packed with spinach, avocado, and mango! And you'll only need about 10 minutes to put this delicious breakfast together!

Preparation time: 10 minutes

Cooking time: 0 minutes

Servings: 2

Ingredients:

- 1 cup of fresh strawberries, hulled
- 2 medium ripe bananas (previously sliced and frozen)
- ¼ of ripe avocado (peeled, pitted, and chopped)
- 1 cup of fresh spinach
- 1 cup of fresh kale, trimmed
- 1 tbsp. of flaxseed meal
- 1½ cups of unsweetened almond milk
- ¼ cup of almonds (toasted and chopped)
- ¼ cup of unsweetened coconut, shredded

Directions:

Put all ingredients into a high-speed blender except almonds and coconut. Pulse to smoothen.

Transfer the puree to bowls and serve immediately with almonds and coconut toppings.

Nutrition:

Calories: 352, Fats: 18.6g, Carbs: 45.3g, Sugar: 19.3g, Proteins: 7.9g, Sodium: 168mg

8. Fruity Bowl

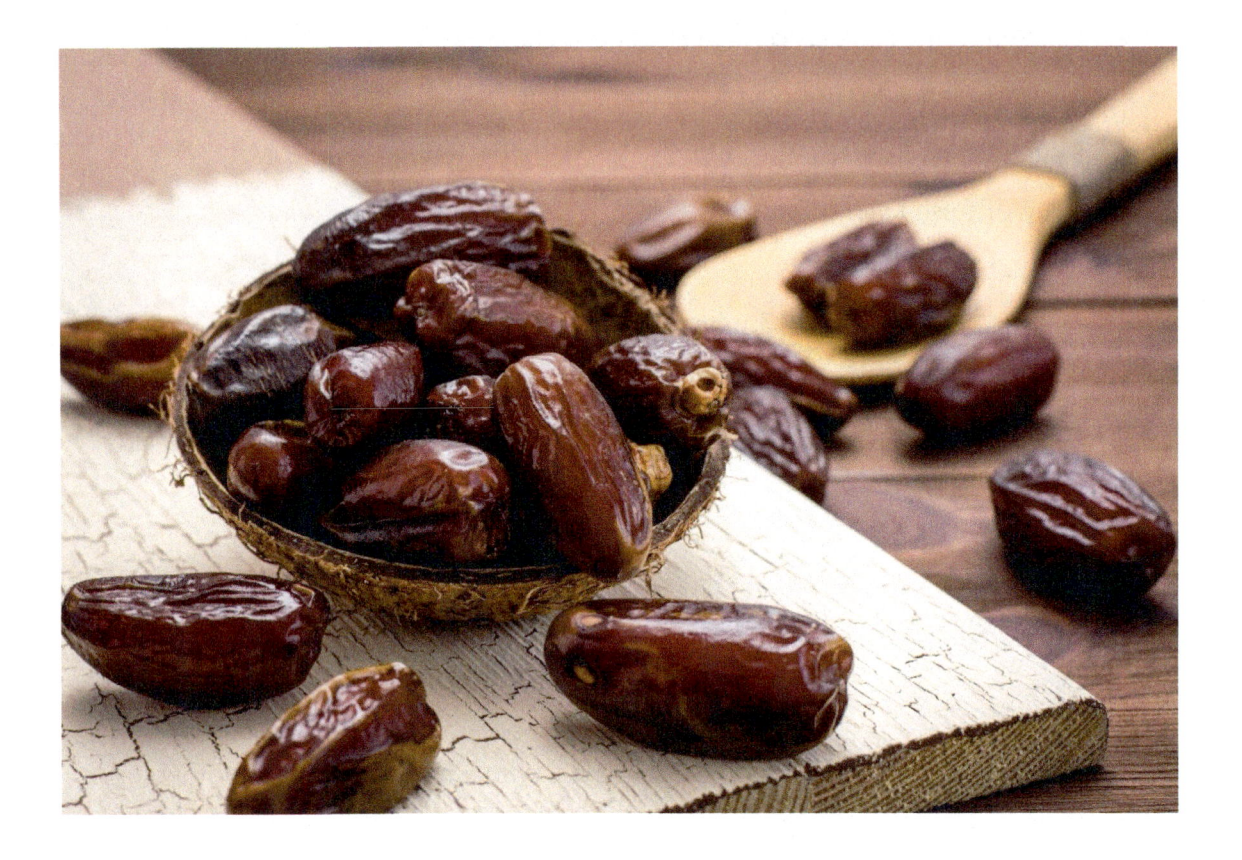

This type of dish is often eaten for breakfast or as a snack. Some people create their own creations to suit their tastes; for example, by using different cereals with different flavors of yogurt and/or fruit.

Preparation time: 10 minutes

Cooking time: 0 minutes

Servings: 2

Ingredients:

- 2 cups of frozen cherries (pitted)
- 4 dates (pitted and chopped)
- 1 large apple (peeled, cored, and chopped)
- A cup of fresh cherries, pitted
- 2 tbsp of Chia seeds

Directions:

Put frozen cherries and dates in a high-speed blender and pulse.

Mix the chopped apple with fresh cherries and Chia seeds in a bowl.

Add cherry sauce to the puree and stir.

Cover and refrigerate them overnight before serving.

Nutrition:

Calories: 211, Fats: 3.2g, Carbs: 49.7g, Sugar: 35g, Proteins: 3.8g, Sodium: 6mg

9. Golden-Orange Overnight Oats

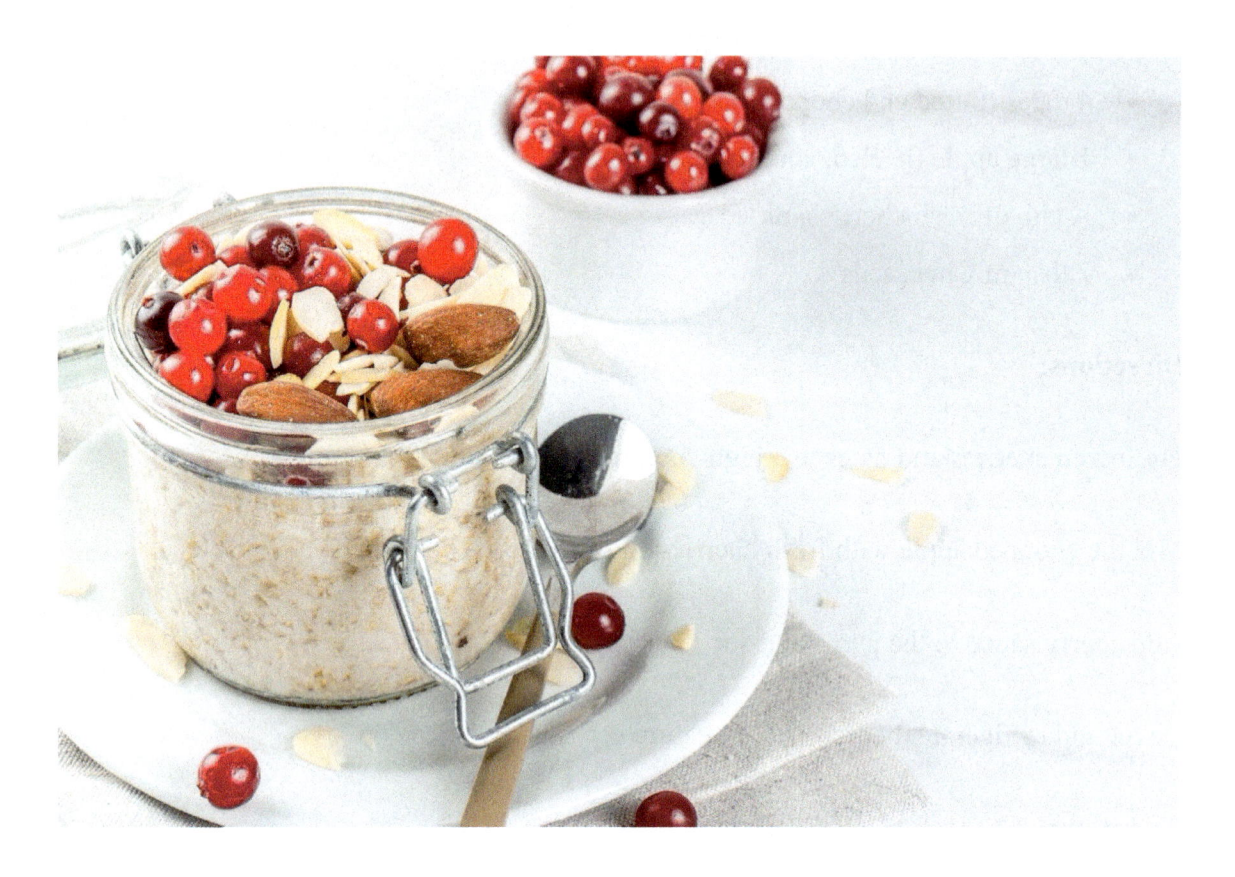

The golden hue of this dish actually comes from turmeric, boosting your levels of anti-inflammatories that are helpful in treating ulcerative colitis. You can top with berries if you want even more healthy, anti-inflammatory compounds in your breakfast.

Preparation Time: 10 minutes + 6-8 hours refrigeration time

Cooking Time: 0 minutes

Servings: 2

Ingredients:

- 1 cup of rolled oats, old-fashioned
- 1 & 1/4 cups of soy milk, vanilla, unsweetened
- 2 tbsp. of syrup, maple
- 1 tsp. of orange zest, fresh
- 3/4 tsp. of turmeric, ground
- 1/4 tsp. of cinnamon, ground
- 1/4 tsp. of salt, kosher
- Optional, for topping: berries, fresh

Directions:

Combine the ingredients except for the berries, if you're using them, in a medium bowl. Combine well. Cover it.

Place in refrigerator for six hours. You can leave it in the fridge overnight if you prefer. Garnish using berries, as desired. Serve.

Nutrition:

Calories: 169 kcal

Protein: 7.14 g

Fat: 4.3 g

Carbohydrates: 38.3 g

10. Banana & Peanut Butter Smoothie

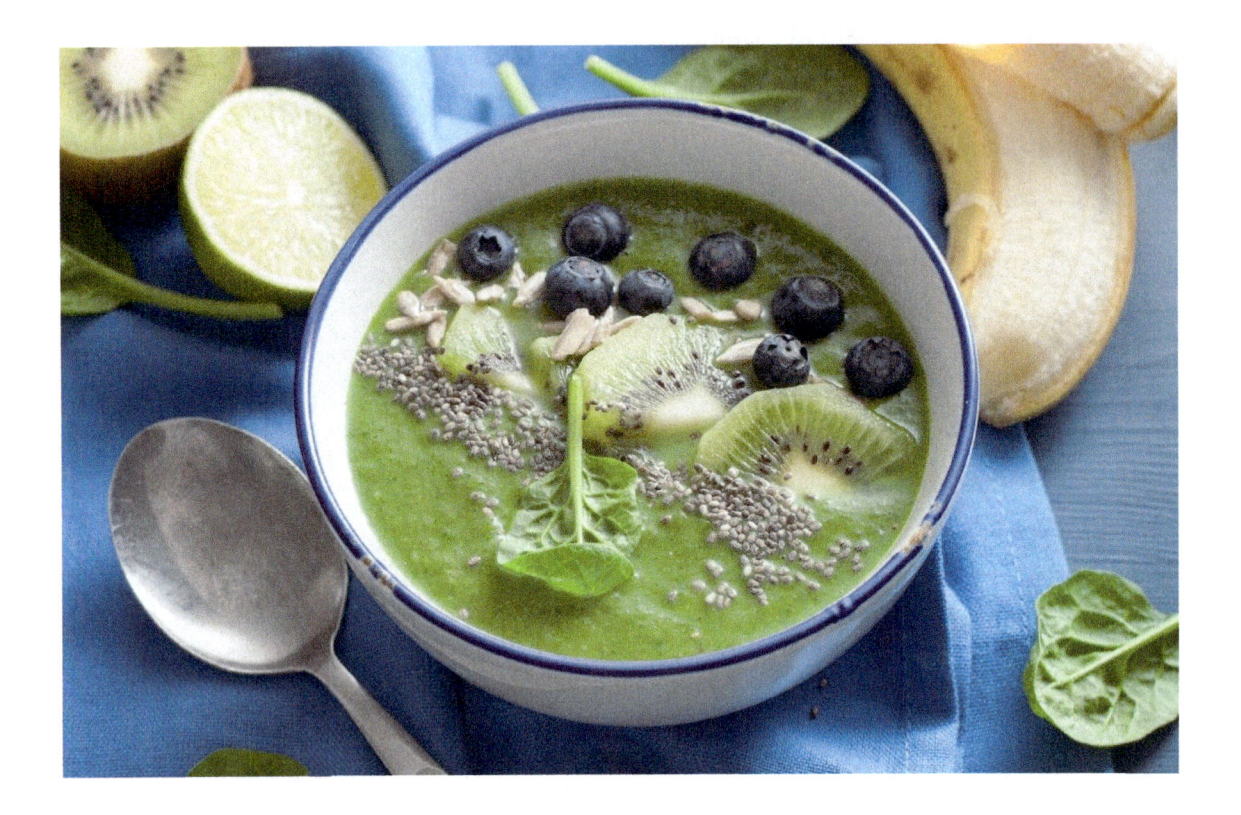

Your body may have difficulty absorbing nutrients if you have ulcerative colitis. This tasty smoothie provides iron and potassium, which your body needs.

Preparation Time: 5 minutes

Cooking Time: 0 minutes

Servings: 1 Serving

Ingredients:

- 1 sliced frozen banana, medium
- 1 cup of spinach, fresh
- 1 cup of soy milk, vanilla, unsweetened
- 1/4 cup of rolled oats, old-fashioned
- 1 tbsp. of peanut butter, natural
- 1/2 tsp. of cinnamon, ground

Directions:

Combine the ingredients in a high-powered food processor.

Blend till fully smooth and serve.

Nutrition:

Calories: 226 kcal

Protein: 10.02 g

Fat: 9.55 g

Carbohydrates: 34.59 g

11. Egg & Sweet Potato Breakfast Hash

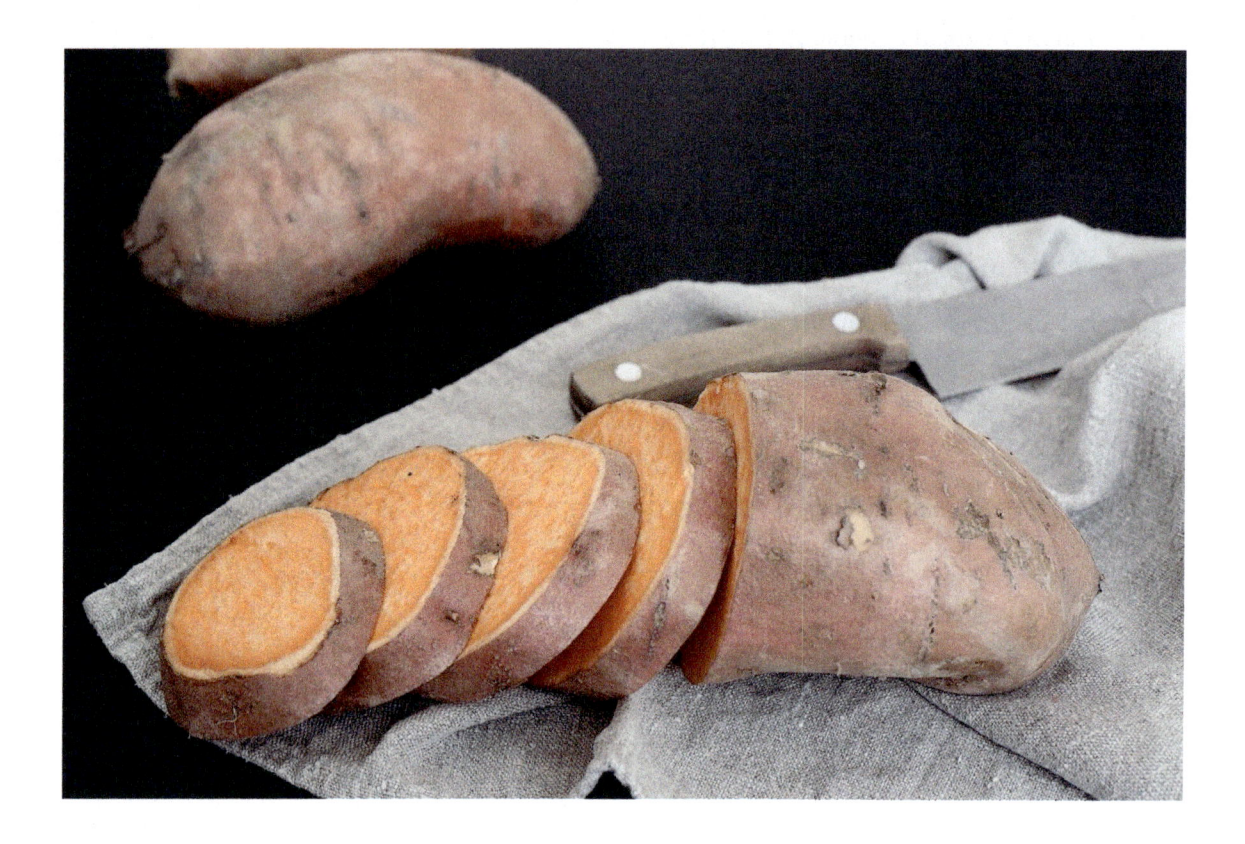

Breakfast hash is an excellent way to increase your intake of veggies. This recipe uses red bell peppers and sweet potatoes for plenty of vitamin A since lots of ulcerative colitis patients lack a healthy vitamin A level.

Preparation Time: 10 minutes

Cooking Time: 20 minutes

Servings: 2

Ingredients:

- 2 & 1/2 tbsp. of oil, olive
- 2 cups of sweet potato, peeled, cubed
- 3/4 cup of chopped bell pepper, red
- 1/4 cup of finely chopped onion, red
- 1/2 tsp. of salt, kosher
- 1/4 tsp. of cumin, ground
- 1/2 tsp. of chili powder
- 2 eggs, large
- 4 tbsp. of salsa, prepared
- 1/2 sliced avocado, ripe
- Optional for garnishing: cilantro, fresh

Directions:

Heat a tbsp. of oil in a large-sized skillet on med. Heat. Add the sweet potatoes. Cook till light gold, four to five minutes.

Add 3 tbsp. of water. Cover skillet. Cook till sweet potatoes become tender while occasionally stirring for seven to eight minutes more.

Add a tbsp. of oil, onions, and bell peppers to the same skillet. Leave uncovered and cook for five minutes or so, till veggies become tender.

Season the hash with 1/4 tsp. of salt, cumin, and chili powder. Transfer to two plates.

Add last 1/2 tsp. of oil to skillet. Crack the eggs into it. Cook for three to four minutes till the whites have set. Season with the last 1/4 tsp. of kosher salt.

Place an egg atop each plate of hash. Top with avocado slices, cilantro, and salsa. Serve.

Nutrition:

Calories: 330 kcal

Protein: 10.34 g

Fat: 26.6 g

Carbohydrates: 20.41 g

12. Apple & Banana Pancakes

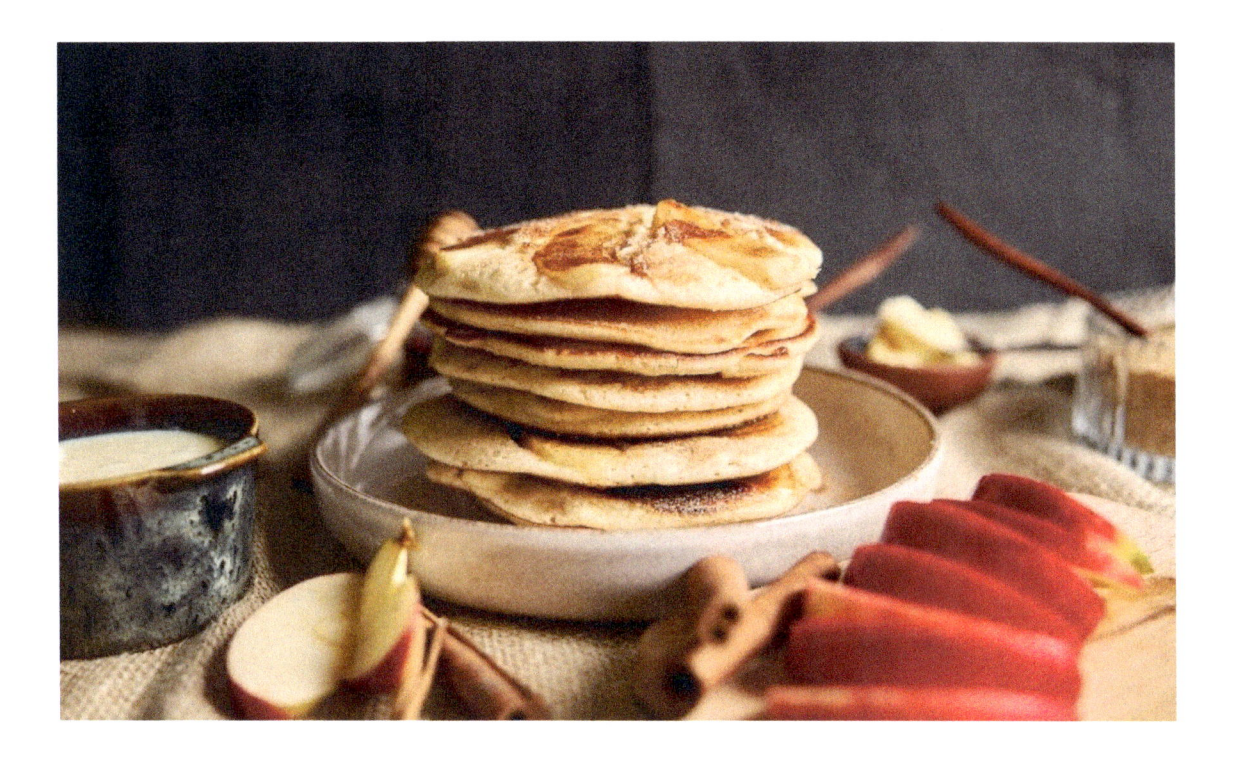

These pancakes offer you the best of both worlds. They're a sweet breakfast treat with no dairy or gluten.

Preparation Time: 10 minutes

Cooking Time: 10 minutes

Servings: 4

Ingredients:

- 6 eggs, small
- 3 bananas, ripe
- 1 apple, grated
- 1 tbsp. of oil, coconut
- Optional: honey, pure

Directions:

Peel bananas. Mash in a medium bowl with a fork.

Core apple. Grate into banana mixture.

Crack eggs into the bowl from step 1. Mix everything together well.

Heat two frying pans. Add a bit of oil to both.

Spoon mixture into pan. Each pan should hold three or four pancakes. Flatten with the back of a spoon, so they're round and thin.

Allow pancakes to cook for one minute till they become golden brown in color on one side. They should be easy to flip with your spatula. Turn pancakes. Allow cooking till another side is golden brown, too.

Once you have cooked the pancakes, remove them from pans. Cook remainder of mixture till gone. Serve pancakes with honey.

Nutrition:

Calories: 248 kcal

Protein: 13.57 g

Fat: 17.94 g

Carbohydrates: 7.81 g

Mains

13. Curried Chicken 'n Rice

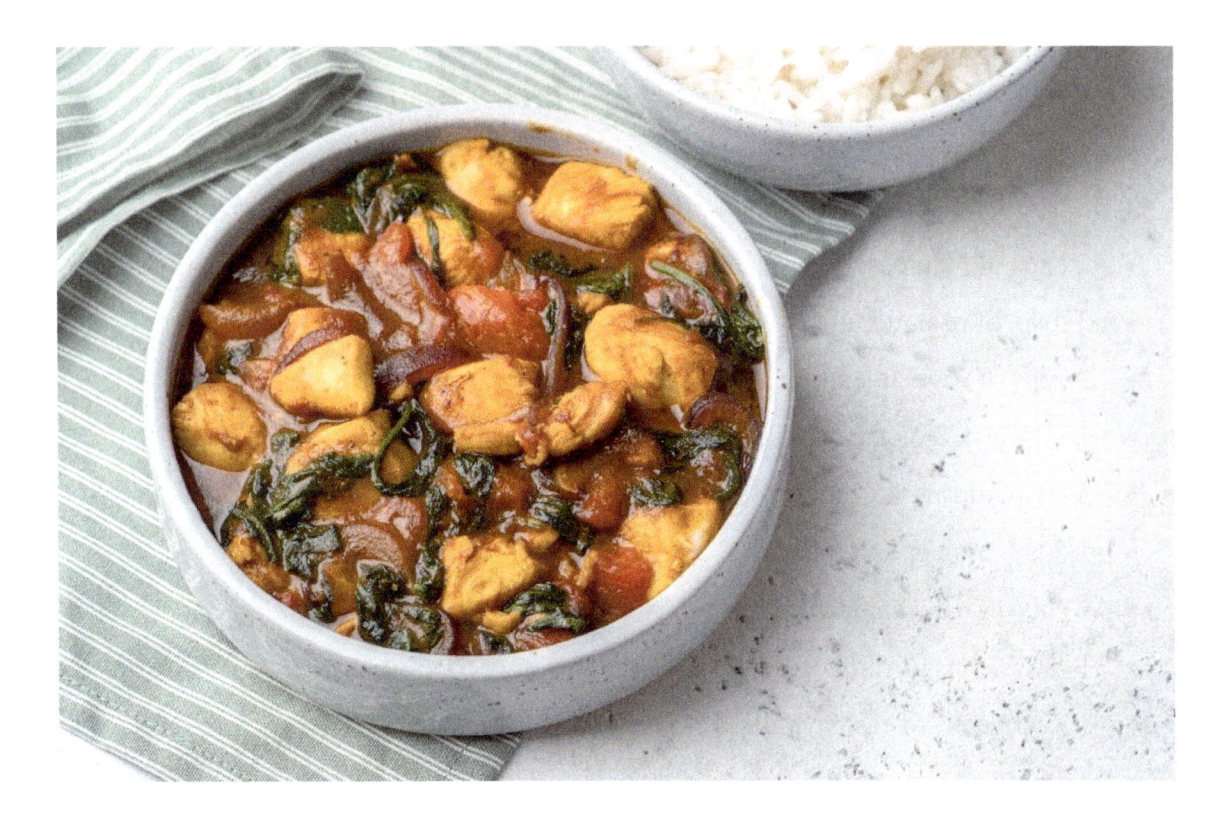

You can actually boost the flavor of a dish by using mild spice blends like the one in this recipe. Shredded meat from chicken breasts is easy on the digestive tract as well.

Preparation Time: 10 minutes

Cooking Time: 30 minutes

Servings: 6

Ingredients:

- 2 tbsp. of oil, olive
- 1 tbsp. of curry powder
- 1 tsp. of paprika, ground
- 2 tsp. of ginger, freshly grated
- 2 cups of potatoes, peeled, cubed
- 3 tbsp. of peanut butter, natural
- 2 cups of vegetable broth, low sodium
- 1 x 14 & 1/2-ounce can of tomatoes, diced
- 3/4 tsp. of salt, kosher
- 1/2 tsp. of pepper, ground
- 2 cups of baby spinach, fresh
- 1 & 1/2 cups of rotisserie chicken, shredded
- 1 & 1/2 cups of cashew milk, refrigerated, unsweetened
- To serve: 3 cups of white rice, cooked
- For garnishing: basil, fresh, as desired

Directions:

Heat the oil in a large skillet on med. Heat it. Add the ginger, curry powder & paprika and cook for two minutes. Stir in the potatoes and occasionally stir for five minutes, till light golden in color.

Add the broth, peanut butter, tomatoes, kosher salt & ground pepper. Bring to boil. Reduce heat level to med-low. Cover skillet and simmer for 18-20 minutes, till potatoes become tender.

Stir in the spinach. Cook for two minutes or so till it wilts. Add cashew milk and chicken. Stir, combining well. Leave uncovered and simmer for five minutes.

Place 1/2 cup of rice each in six bowls. Top with a cup of curry mixture. Use basil to garnish, as desired. Serve.

Nutrition:

Calories: 240 kcal

Protein: 6.04 g

Fat: 9.3 g

Carbohydrates: 33.73 g

14. Rice Noodles & Tofu

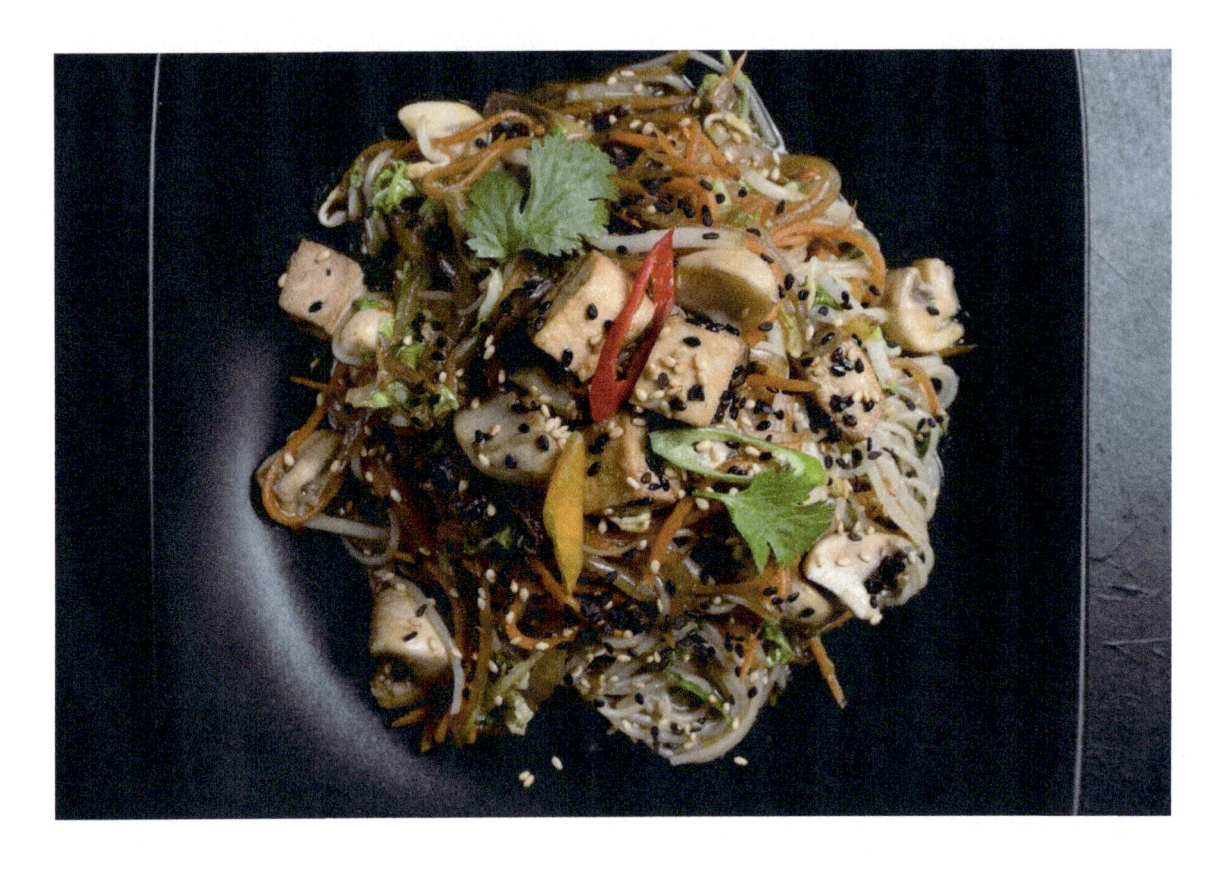

You can lower your inflammation levels by eating a diet that is more plant-based. Using tofu and frozen veggies makes this dish easy to prepare, too.

Preparation Time: 20 minutes

Cooking Time: 30 minutes

Servings: 2

Ingredients:

- 1 tbsp. of oil, sesame
- 1 tbsp. of peanut butter, smooth, all-natural
- 1 tbsp. of syrup, maple
- 3 tbsp. of soy sauce, reduced-sodium
- 2 tbsp. of lime juice, fresh
- 1 x 8-ounce block of tofu, organic, extra firm
- 2 tsp. of oil, sesame
- 2 cups of vegetables, frozen, like water chestnuts, bell peppers, green beans, carrots, etc.
- Optional: 1 can of corn, rinsed
- 6 ounces of noodles, rice
- Optional: cilantro, fresh

Directions:

Preheat oven to 400F.

Cut the tofu into small cubes.

Whisk the first five ingredients together. Toss with the tofu.

Spread tofu on a lined cookie sheet. Bake in 400F oven for 20-25 minutes.

Cook the noodles using directions on the package.

Heat 2 tsp. oil in a large-sized pan. Sauté veggies till they become tender.

Split the noodles into two bowls. Top with vegetables and tofu. Add cilantro and serve.

Nutrition:

Calories: 285 kcal

Protein: 6.51 g

Fat: 9.71 g

Carbohydrates: 47.1 g

15. Chicken & Cheese Pasta Salad

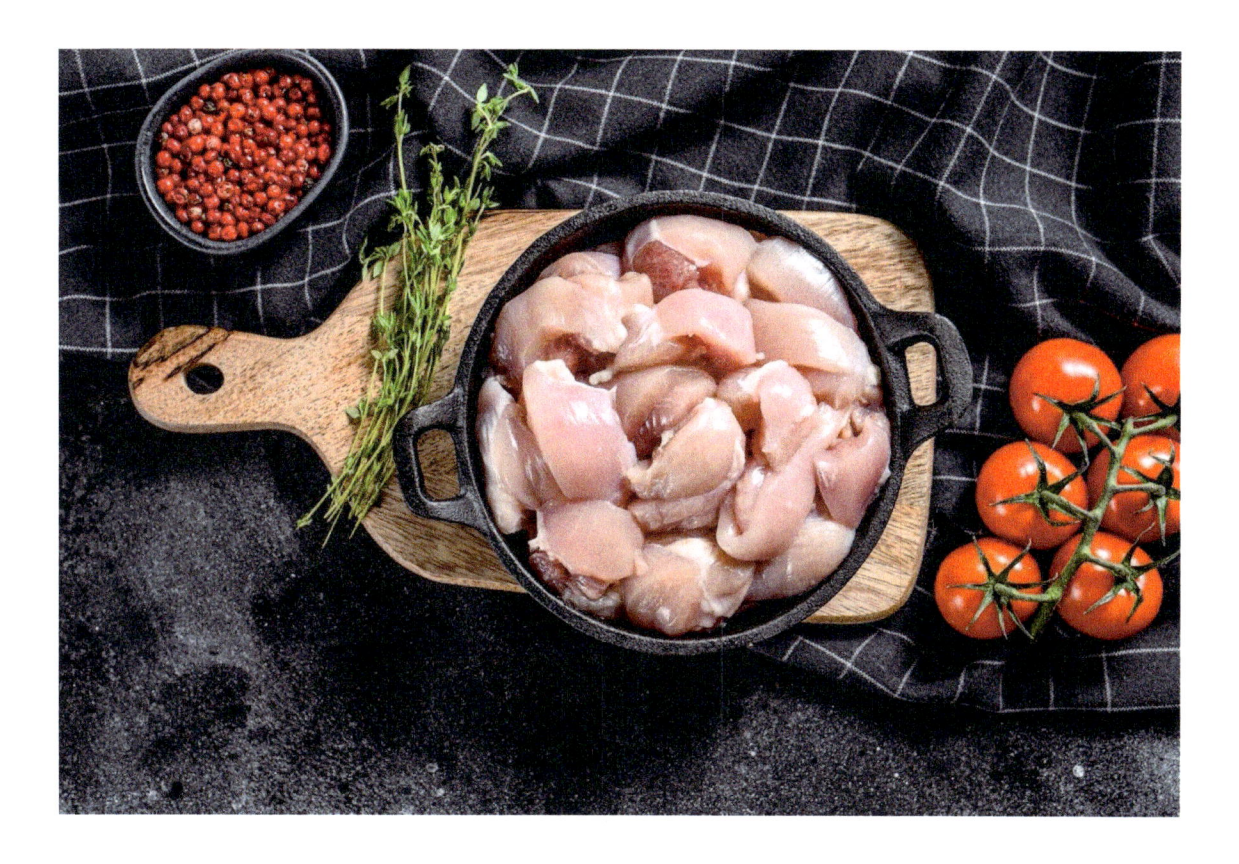

If you have UC and eat a Mediterranean diet, the food fights inflammation and can allow you to have fewer flare-ups. This salad offers a great taste with vegetables and lean protein.

Preparation Time: 15 minutes

Cooking Time: 20 minutes

Servings: 6

Ingredients:

- 1 pound of chicken breasts, skinless, boneless
- 1 tsp. of salt, kosher
- 1/2 tsp. of pepper, black
- 1/2 tsp. of paprika, ground
- Non-stick spray
- 12 ounces of pasta, rotini or fusilli, dry
- 2 tsp. of minced garlic, fresh
- 2 tsp. of mustard, Dijon
- 1 tbsp. of chopped oregano, fresh
- 2 tbsp. of vinegar, red wine
- 1/4 cup of oil, olive
- 4 cups of baby spinach, fresh
- 1 pint of halved tomatoes, cherry
- 1 x 14-ounce can of drained artichoke hearts
- 1 x 2 & 1/4-ounce can of drained black olives, sliced
- Optional: 1/2 cup of feta cheese, crumbled

Directions:

Evenly season the chicken using 1/2 tsp. of salt, pepper & ground paprika.

Heat grill pan on med-high. Coat pan and meat using non-stick spray. Add the chicken. Cook for five minutes per side or till done. Remove the chicken from its pan. Allow standing for five minutes. Slice in small pieces.

Cook pasta using directions on the package. Drain. Rinse using cold water—place in a large-sized bowl.

As pasta is cooking, combine the vinegar, oregano, mustard, garlic, and last 1/2 tsp. of salt in a medium bowl. Whisk and stir well. Gradually stream in the oil while continuously whisking, till combined well.

Add artichokes, tomatoes, spinach, and olives in a bowl with the pasta. Toss and combine. Add the chicken, then feta, and the dressing. Combine well. Serve.

Nutrition:

Calories: 335 kcal

Protein: 20.03 g

Fat: 20.07 g

Carbohydrates: 18.94 g

16. Tasty Salmon Burger

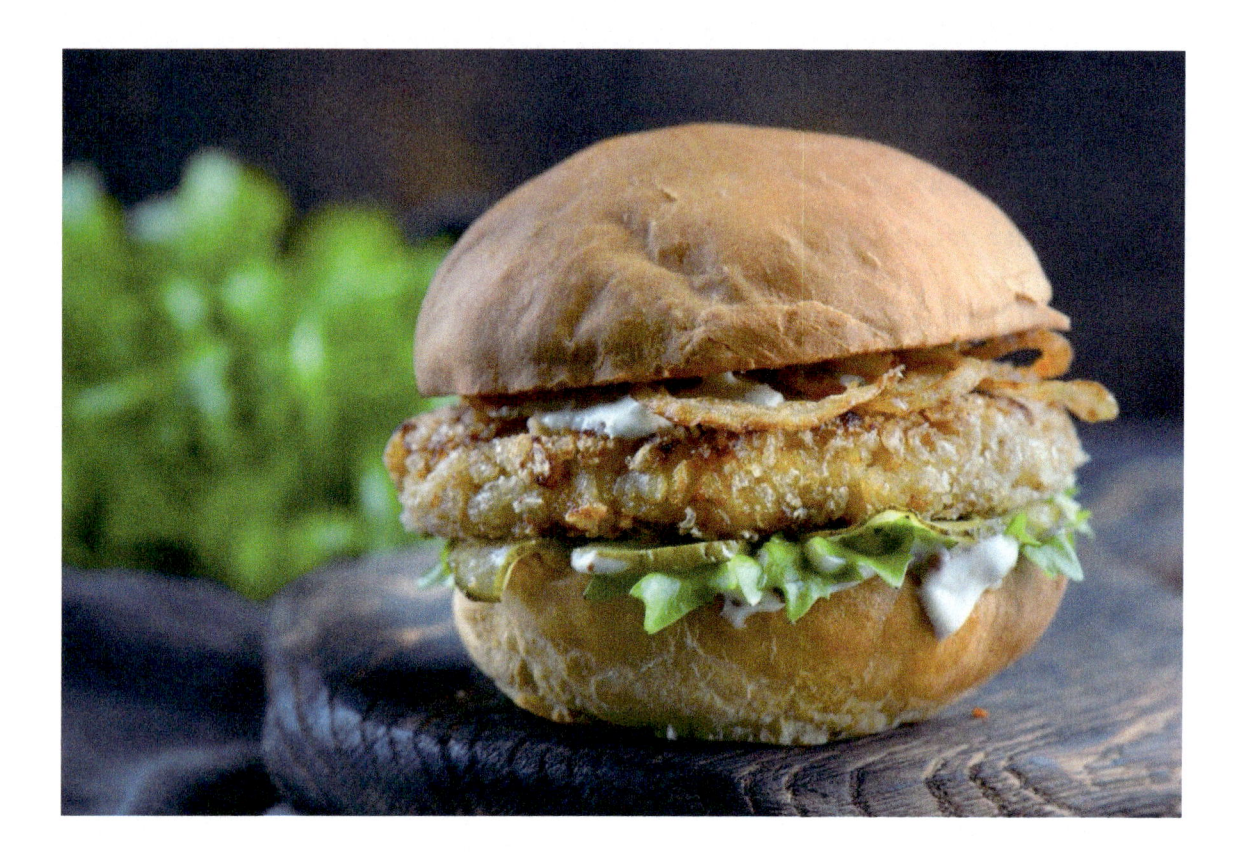

Canned salmon is easy to cook with, and it provides your body with omega-3 fats, which can help in reducing inflammation. You'll love it for lunch or dinner.

Preparation Time: 10 minutes

Cooking Time: 10 minutes

Servings: 5

Ingredients:

- 1 egg, large
- 1 x 14 & 3/4-ounce can of salmon
- 1/2 cup of breadcrumbs, gluten-free
- 1 tbsp. of oil, olive

Directions:

Mix the ingredients together in a medium or large bowl.

Shape mixture in five patties.

Add the oil to a large skillet on med. Heat. Cook salmon patties for a few minutes per side till they have browned. Serve.

Nutrition:

Calories: 70 kcal

Protein: 3.2 g

Fat: 5.12 g

Carbohydrates: 2.68 g

17. Roast Tarragon Chicken

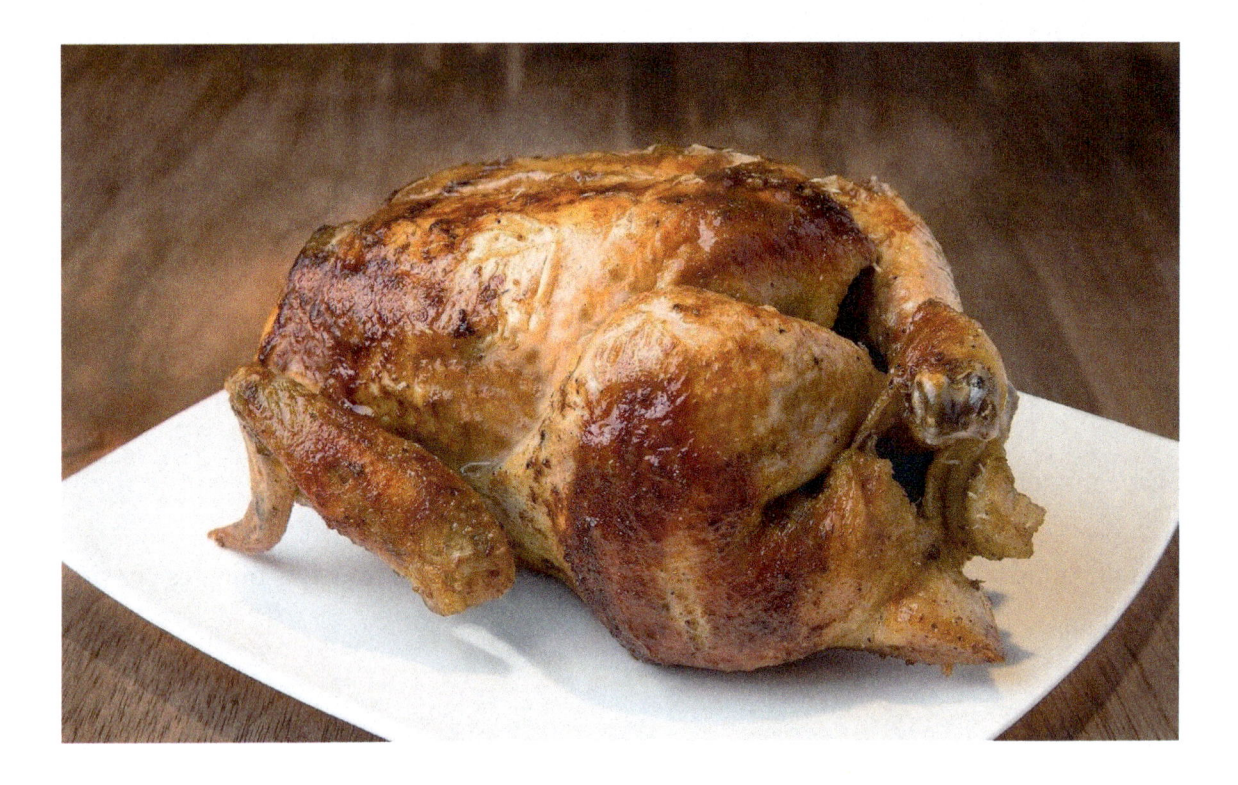

Roast chicken doesn't need to be fussed over or cooked using complicated techniques. In making UC dishes, sometimes simpler is better.

Preparation Time: 30 minutes

Cooking Time: 2 hours **and 20 minutes**

Servings: 8

Ingredients:

- 1 peeled, quartered onion, small
- 3 peeled, quartered garlic cloves
- 1/4 tsp. of tarragon, powdered
- 1/4 tsp. of thyme, powdered
- 1 x 5-pound chicken – remove the giblets
- 2 tbsp. of oil, olive
- 1 tsp. of salt, kosher

Directions:

Preheat the oven to 375F.

Place garlic, onions, thyme and tarragon powders in the chicken cavity. Tie legs together using string and close the opening of the cavity. Pull wings till tips overlap atop breast and tie them in place.

Rub chicken with salt and oil and set it in a roast pan with the breast side facing down.

Roast the chicken for 25 minutes on one side. Turn with the breast side facing up. Continue to roast and occasionally baste with juices from the pan, till internal temp is 175F, an hour & 15 minutes to an hour & 1/2.

Transfer the chicken to the cutting board. Allow resting for 8-10 minutes. Remove string and carve. Serve.

Nutrition:

Calories: 109 kcal

Protein: 10.54 g

Fat: 6.35 g

Carbohydrates: 2.01 g

18. Niçoise Lettuce-Free "Salad"

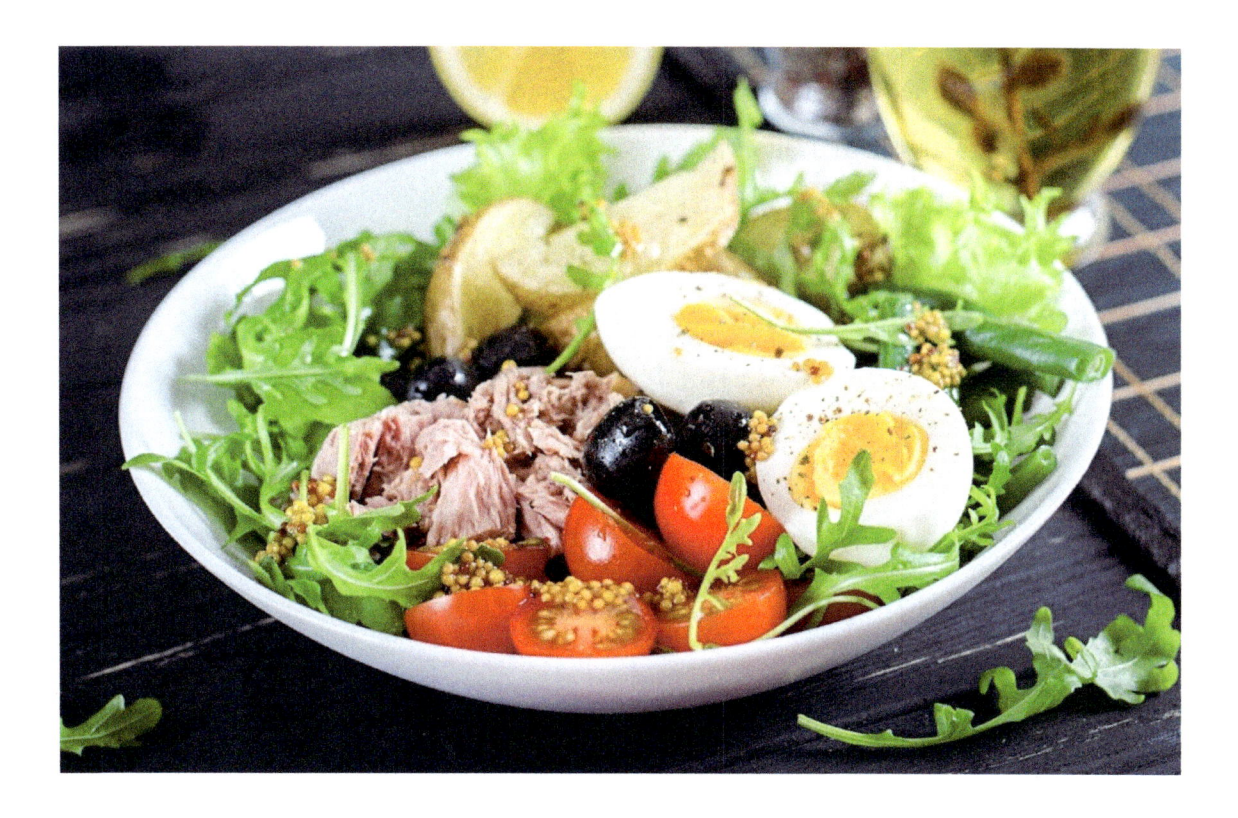

Traditional salads are not usually acceptable fare for people with ulcerative colitis. This "salad" has no lettuce, so you get the flavor without the excess roughage you don't need.

Preparation Time: 15 minutes

Cooking Time: 0 minutes

Servings: 1-2

Ingredients:

- 2 chopped eggs, hard-boiled
- 1 x 5 or 6-ounce can of drained tuna packed in water
- 1 halved, chopped avocado, ripe
- 12 halved olives, Kalamata
- 3 tbsp. of oil, olive
- Salt, sea, as desired
- Optional: Pepper, black, as desired
- 3 to 4 tsp. of dill, dried

Directions:

Prepare ingredients as listed above.

Combine the eggs through the olives in a large-sized bowl and toss with oil.

Season as desired and serve.

Nutrition:

Calories: 424 kcal

Protein: 20.71 g

Fat: 35.04 g

Carbohydrates: 8.84 g

19. Spaghetti Squash Boats

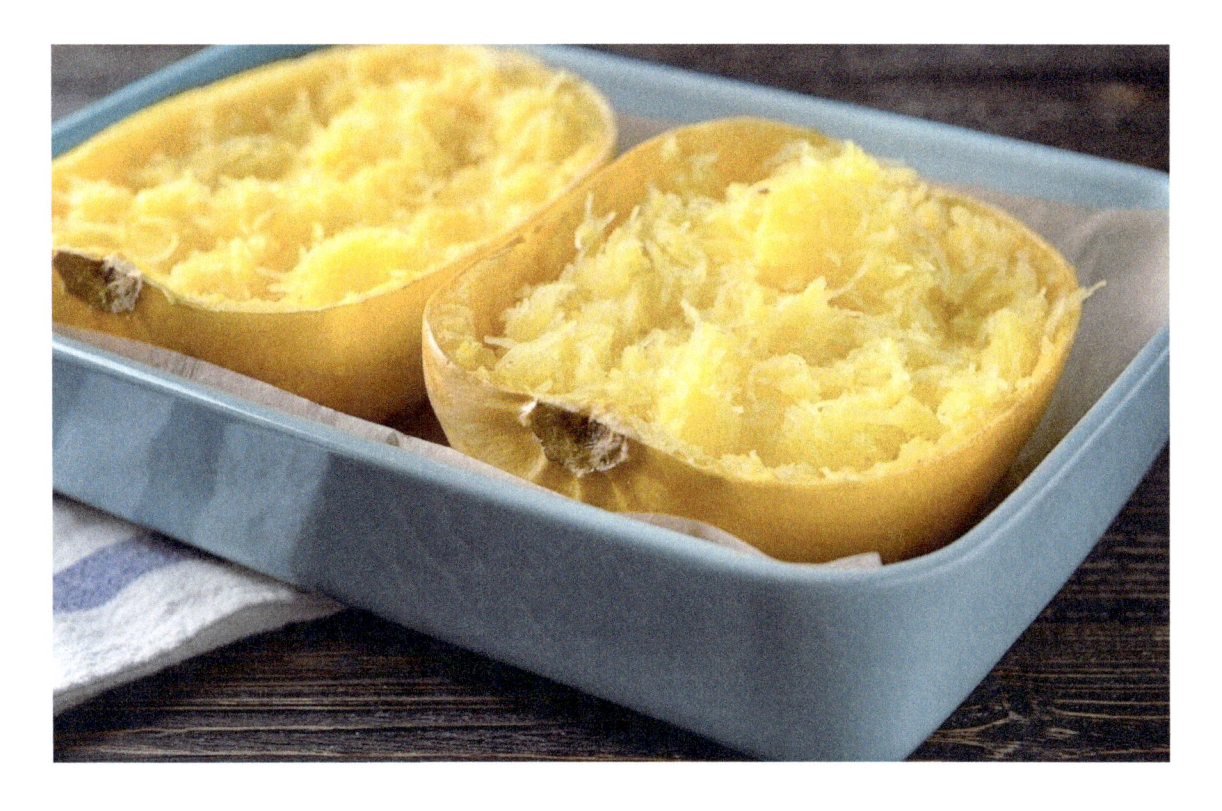

Traditional filled squash boats may include dairy produce and ground beef, which can exacerbate your UC symptoms. Instead, try faux cheese and lean turkey, as this recipe uses.

Preparation Time: 15 minutes

Cooking Time: 40 minutes

Servings: 4

Ingredients:

- 2 spaghetti squash, medium
- 2 tbsp. of oil, olive
- 1 pound of turkey breast, ground
- 2 cups of baby spinach, fresh
- 3/4 tsp. of salt, kosher
- 1 x 15-ounce can of tomatoes, crushed
- 4 tbsp. of basil leaves, chopped, fresh
- 3/4 cup of almonds, blanched
- 2 tsp. of lemon juice, fresh
- 1 tsp. of yeast, nutritional
- 1/3 cup of water, warm

Directions:

Preheat the oven to 400F.

Slice squash lengthwise in halves. Remove & discard seeds. Brush the flesh using 1 tbsp. oil. Place on a rimmed cookie sheet with the cut side facing down.

Bake in 400F oven for 35-40 minutes, till flesh becomes fork-tender.

Heat last tbsp. oil in a large-sized skillet on med. Heat. Add the turkey and break apart while you cook till it is done through six to seven minutes.

Add spinach and stir. Cook till it wilts, two minutes. Season it using 1/2 tsp. of kosher salt.

Add tomatoes and stir. Add 2 tbsp. of basil and stir again. Reduce the heat level to low. Cover skillet and keep the mixture warm.

Combine water, yeast, lemon juice, almonds, and last 1/4 tsp. of kosher salt in a blender and blend till smooth.

Remove the squash from the oven. Shred flesh into strands like spaghetti. Evenly fill squash halves with the turkey and vegetable mixture. Top with 2 tbsp. of almond-based ricotta. Evenly garnish with the last tbsp. of basil and serve.

Nutrition:

Calories: 249 kcal

Protein: 25.8 g

Fat: 14.97 g

Carbohydrates: 1.61 g

20. Chicken Piccata on Pasta

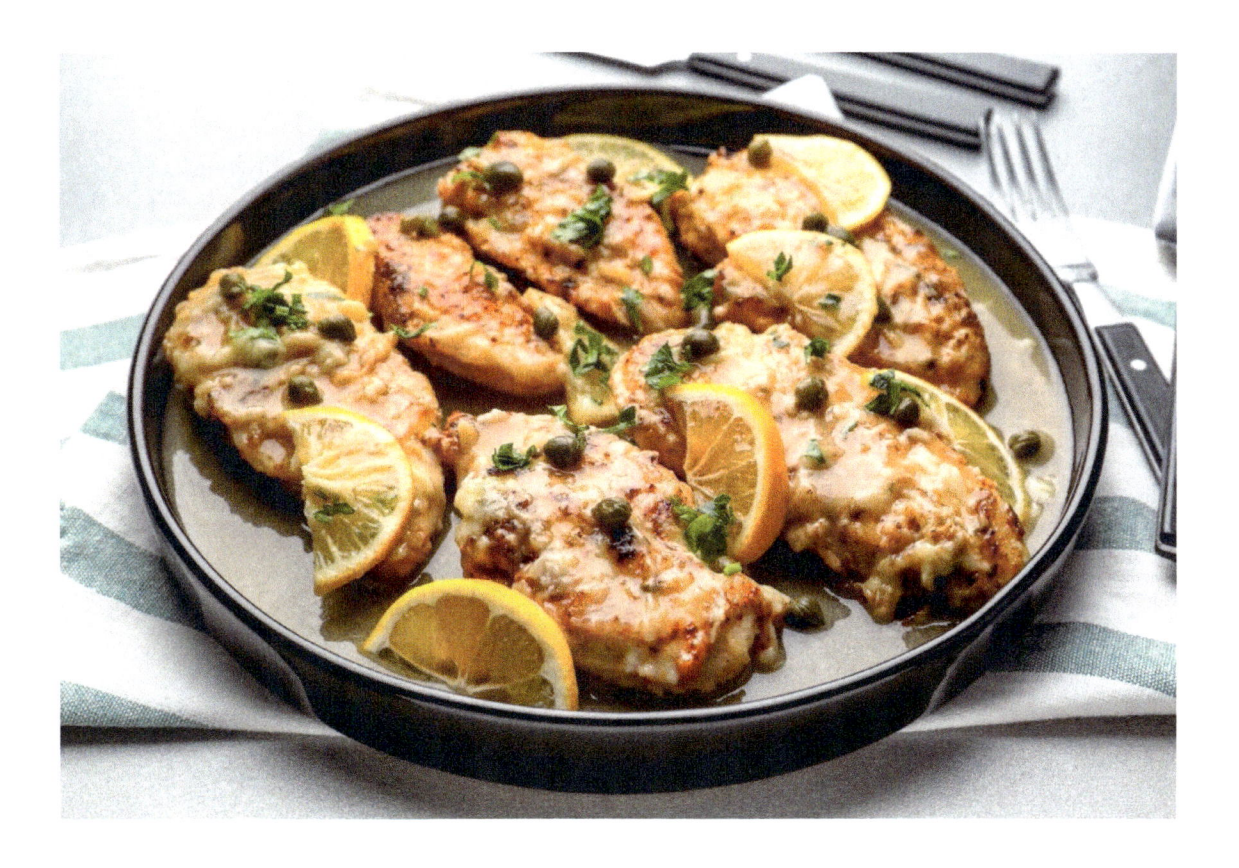

This pasta dish uses less butter, so it doesn't include much-saturated fat, which could otherwise be a trigger for your ulcerative colitis. Add a boost of antioxidants by including capers in the dish.

Preparation Time: 15 minutes

Cooking Time: 20 minutes

Servings: 4

Ingredients:

- 10 ounces of pasta, angel hair, dry
- 3 tbsp. of oil, olive
- 3 tbsp. of butter, unsalted
- 1 pound of butterflied, halved chicken breasts, boneless, skinless
- 1/2 tsp. of salt, kosher
- 3/4 tsp. of pepper, black
- 3 tbsp. of flour, all-purpose
- 1 tsp. of minced garlic, fresh
- 1/2 cup of dry wine, white
- 1 cup of chicken broth, low sodium
- 2 tbsp. of lemon juice, fresh
- 1/4 cup of drained capers, brined
- 1/3 cup of chopped parsley, fresh

Directions:

Cook the pasta using directions on the package. Drain. Add to a serving platter.

Heat 2 tbsp. butter and oil in a large-sized skillet on med-high. Season the chicken as desired. Evenly coat in flour and shake off the excess.

Add the chicken to the hot skillet. Cook for three minutes per side without moving it except to turn it, till golden brown in color. Transfer chicken to plate.

Add the garlic to the skillet. Stir constantly while cooking for a minute. Then, add the wine and cook for two minutes. Scrape up any brown bits from the pan till the liquid has been reduced by about half.

Add and stir broth, capers, lemon juice & 1/4 tsp. pepper. Add the chicken back into the pan. Simmer for five minutes.

Remove the chicken from the skillet. Place atop pasta. Add the last tbsp. butter to skillet. Vigorously whisk and combine well.

Pour the sauce over the chicken & pasta. Use fresh parsley to garnish and serve.

Nutrition:

Calories: 493 kcal

Protein: 35.8 g

Fat: 25.76 g

Carbohydrates: 30.24 g

21. Turkey with Thyme & Sage Sausage

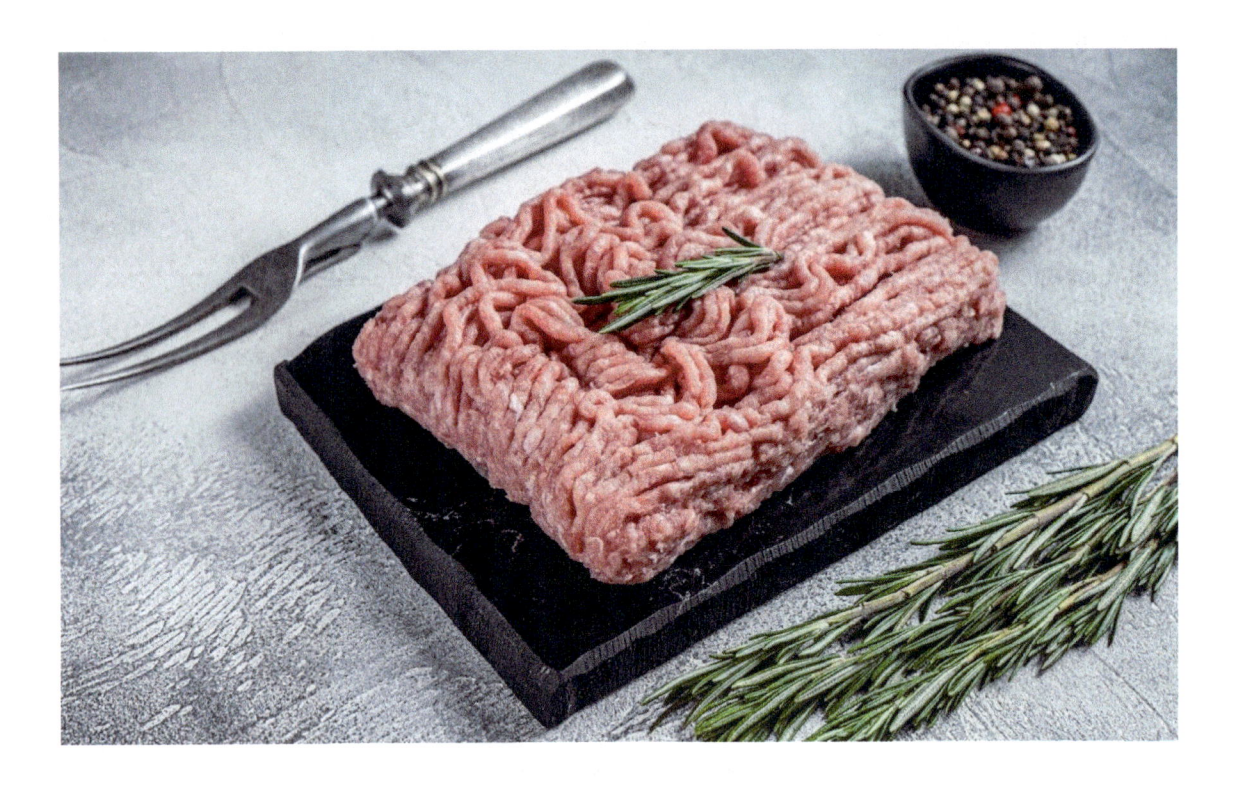

This dish is a variation of a traditional turkey breast stuffing that replaces bread with ground pork sausage. Sage and thyme are the signature flavors in the recipe, as they give the dish an earthy taste for a Thanksgiving-worthy meal.

Preparation Time: 40-minutes

Cooking Time: 25-minutes

Servings: 4

Ingredients:

- 1 lb. ground turkey
- ½ tsp. cinnamon
- ½ tsp. garlic powder
- 1 tsp. fresh rosemary
- 1 tsp. fresh thyme
- 1 tsp. sea salt
- 2 tsp. fresh sage
- 2 tbsp. coconut oil

Directions:

Stir in all the ingredients, except for the oil, in a mixing bowl. Refrigerate overnight or for 30 minutes.

Pour the oil into the mixture. Form the mixture into four patties.

In a lightly greased skillet placed over medium heat, cook the patties for 5 minutes on each side or until their middle portions are no longer pink. You can also cook them by baking in the oven for 25 minutes at 400°F.

Nutrition: Calories: 284 Fat: 9.4g Protein: 14.2g Sodium: 290mg Total Carbs: 36.9g Dietary Fiber: 0.7g Net Carbs: 36.2g

22. Blackened Chicken Breast

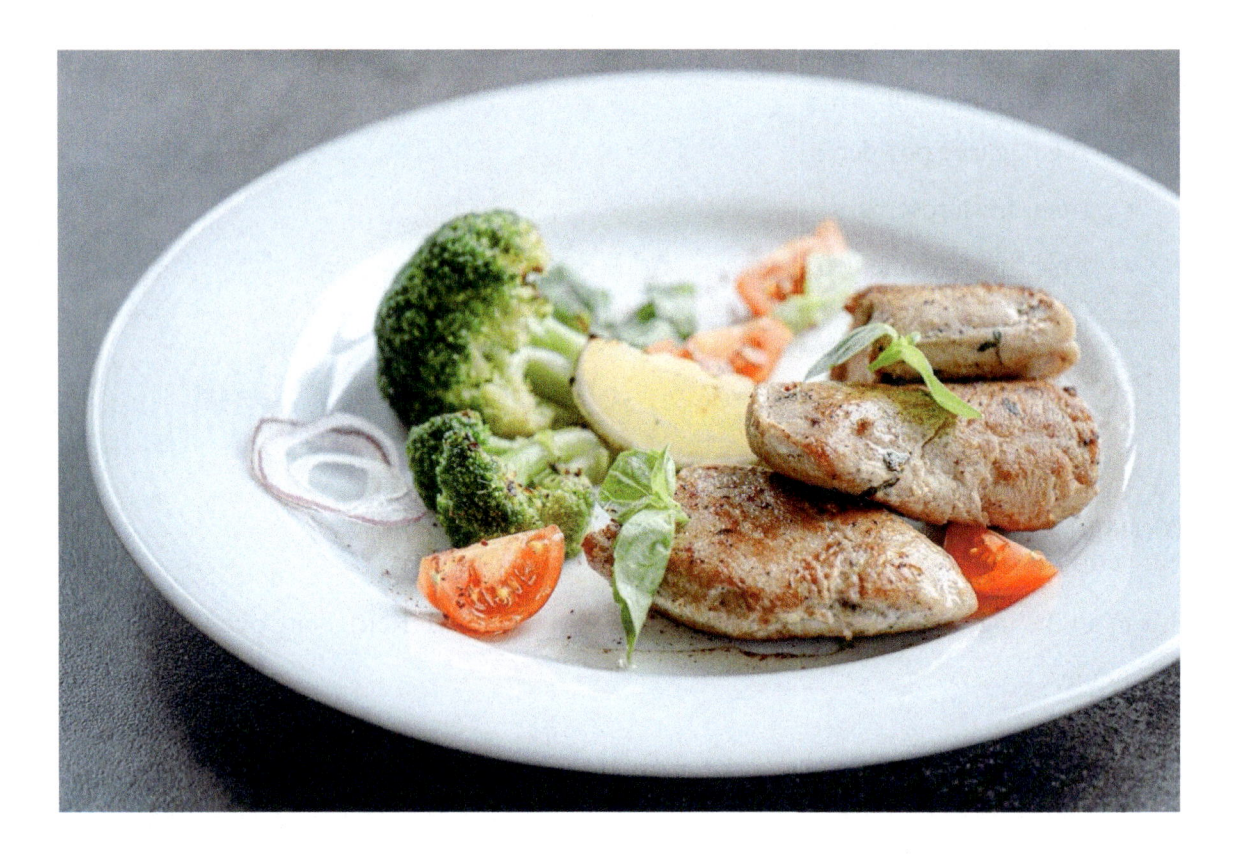

For this recipe, chicken breasts are seasoned and then cooked in a cast-iron skillet for good char. It is a classic dish that can be found on any authentic Cajun menu.

Preparation Time: 10 minutes

Cooking Time: 15 minutes

Servings: 2

Ingredients:

- chicken breast halves, skinless and boneless
- 1 tsp. thyme, ground
- 2 tsp. of paprika
- 2 tsp. olive oil
- 1 tsp. salt
- ½ tsp. onion powder

Directions:

Combine the thyme, paprika, onion powder, and salt together in your bowl.

Transfer the spice mix to a flat plate.

Rub olive oil on the chicken breast. Coat fully.

Roll the chicken pieces in the spice mixture. Press down, ensuring that all sides have the spice mix.

Keep aside for 5 minutes.

In the meantime, preheat your air fryer to 360 degrees F.

Keep the chicken in the air fryer basket—Cook for 8 minutes.

Flip once and cook for another 7 minutes.

Transfer the breasts to a serving plate. Serve after 5 minutes.

Nutrition: Calories 424 Carbohydrates 3g Cholesterol 198mg Total Fat 11g Protein 79g Sugar 1g Fiber 2g Sodium 516mg

23. Creamy Pesto Chicken

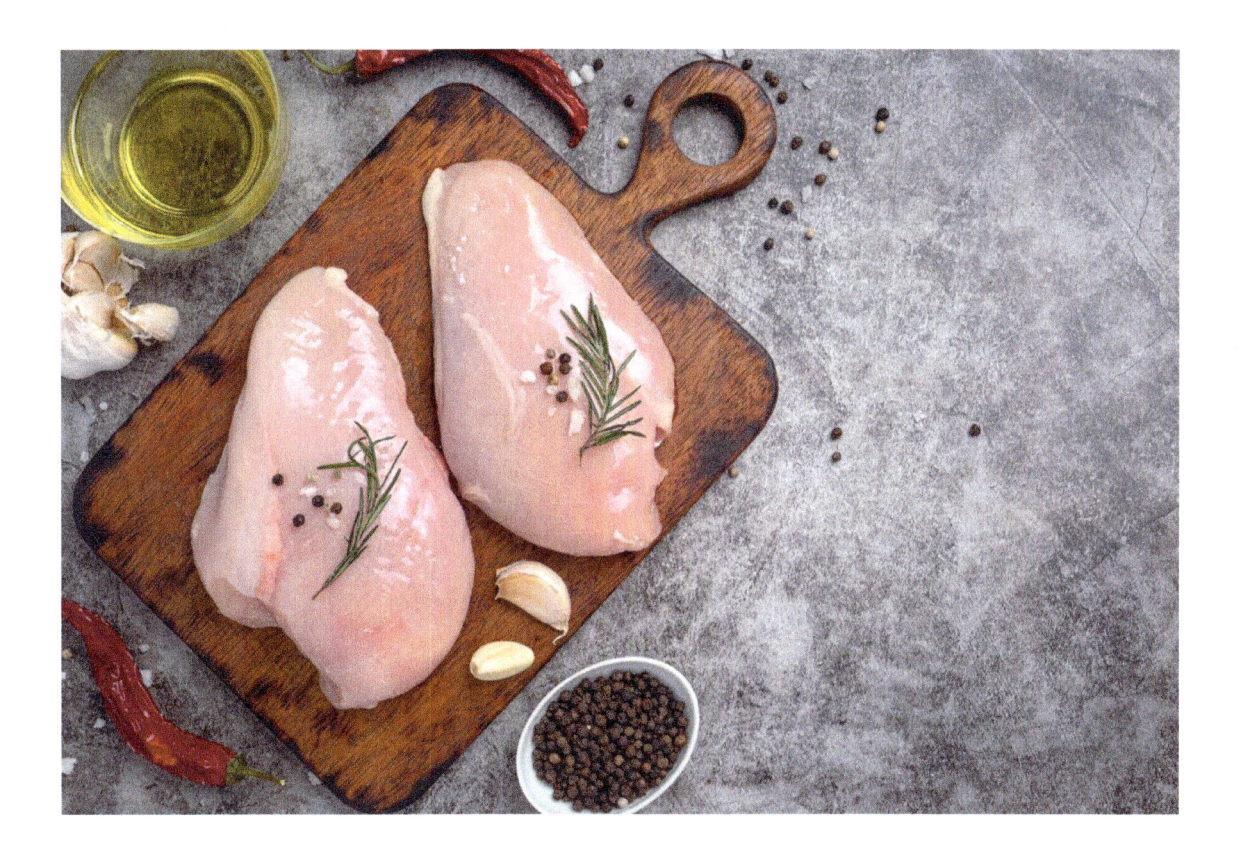

 This Creamy Pesto Chicken recipe is a healthy, delicious meal that can be easily made in one pot. It's the perfect winter meal. This creamy pesto chicken recipe has an easy prep time and comes together in one pot.

Preparation time: 20 minutes

Cooking time: 20 minutes

Servings: 4

Ingredients:

For chicken:

- 2 tbsp. balsamic vinegar
- 2 tsp. dried oregano
- ½ tsp salt or to taste
- 2 tsp. olive oil
- 1 tsp minced garlic
- boneless, skinless, chicken breast halves (6 oz each)

For pesto:

- ½ cup loosely packed basil leaves
- ½ tsp salt
- ½ cup packed fresh parsley leaves
- ½ cup canned coconut milk

Directions:

To make chicken: Combine balsamic vinegar, oregano, salt, olive oil, and garlic in a bowl. Brush this mixture over the chicken and place the chicken in a baking dish that has been sprayed with cooking spray.

To make pesto: Blend together basil, salt, and parsley in the food processor until finely chopped.

With the blender machine running, pour coconut milk through the feeder tube in a thin drizzle until smooth and well combined.

Divide chicken into serving plates. Place 2 tablespoons pesto on each plate and serve.

Nutrition: Calories – 261 Fat – 11 g Total Carbohydrate – 4 g Protein – 35 g

24. Salmon and Dill Pâté

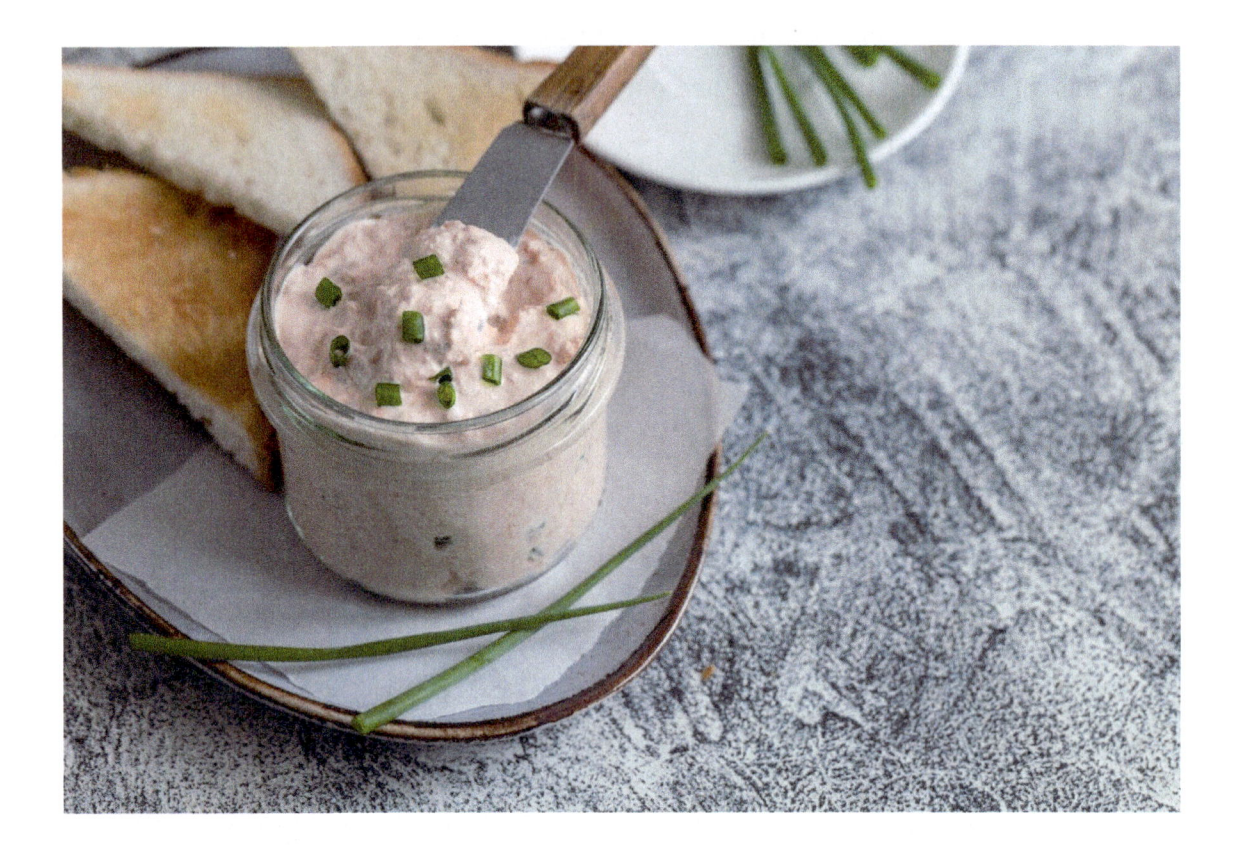

Salmon and Dill Pâté is a delicious, high-protein salmon dip that's low-fat and gluten-free. Salmon is rich in omega 3 fatty acids, which are important for brain development, skin health, heart function, healthy joints, and more!

Preparation Time: 10 Minutes

Cooking Time: 8 Minutes

Servings: 4

Ingredients:

- 6 ounces cooked salmon, bones and skin removed
- ¼ cup heavy (whipping) cream
- 1 tbsp. chopped fresh dill or 1½ teaspoons dried
- zest of 1 lemon
- ½ tsp. sea salt

Directions:

In a blender or food processor (or in a large bowl using a mixer), combine the salmon, lemon zest, heavy cream, dill, and salt. Blend until smooth.

Nutrition: Calories 197 kcal Total Fat 11g Carbs 5g Protein 15g Sugar 2g

25. Vegetable and Chicken Stir Fry

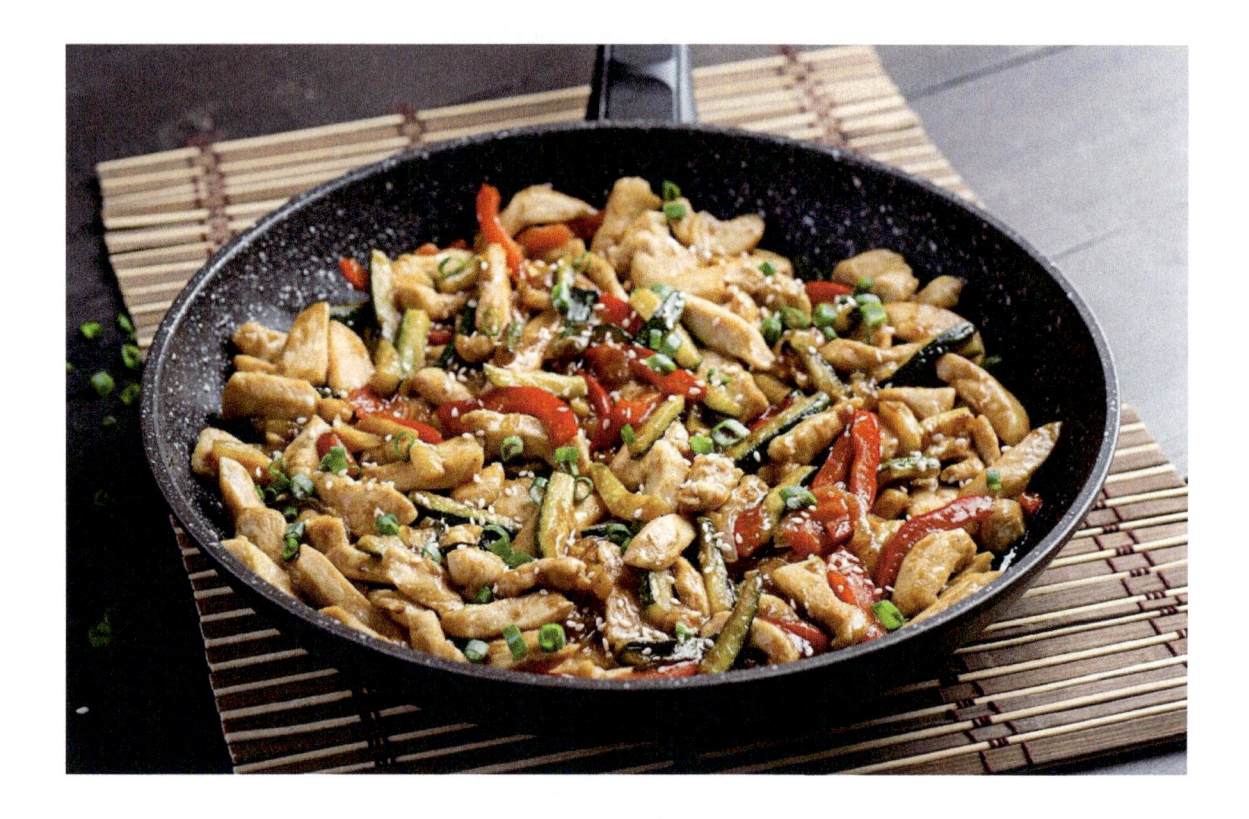

This is a tasty and light meal, ideal for those warm summer evenings where you want something that will make you feel all cool and breezy.

Preparation Time: 5 minutes

Cooking Time: 15 minutes

Servings: 6

Ingredients:

- 1 tbsp. of olive oil
- chicken breasts
- 3 medium zucchini or yellow squash
- 2 onions
- 1 tsp. of garlic powder
- 1 broccoli
- 1 tsp. basil
- 1 tsp. of pepper and salt

Directions:

Chop the vegetables and chicken.

Heat your skillet over medium temperature.

Pour olive oil and add the chicken. Cook while stirring.

Include the seasonings if you want.

Add the vegetables. Keep cooking until it gets slightly soft. Add the onions first and broccoli last.

Nutrition: Calories 183 Carbohydrates 9g Cholesterol 41mg Total Fat 11g Protein 12g Sugar 4g Fiber 3g Sodium 468mg

26. Curried Shrimp and Vegetables

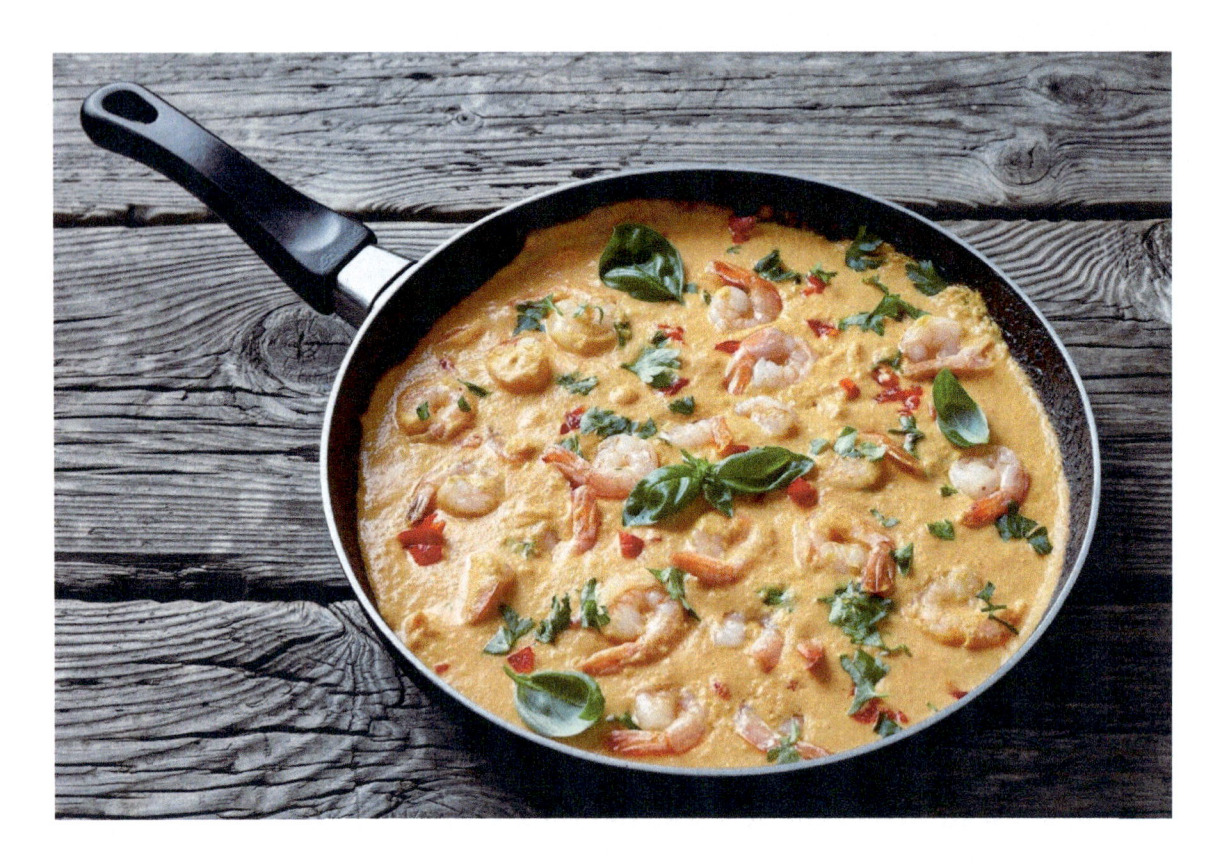

Curried Shrimp and Vegetables is a delicious shrimp dish with sweet potatoes, peas, and coconut milk. Spices like turmeric, cumin, ginger, salt, and pepper are added for flavor. A typical dinner usually calls for rice to go alongside it.

Preparation Time: 10 minutes

Cooking Time: 15 minutes

Servings: 4

Ingredients:

- 3 tbsp. coconut oil
- 1 onion, sliced
- 2 cups cauliflower, cut into florets
- 1 cup of coconut milk
- 1 tbsp. curry powder
- ¼ cup fresh parsley, chopped
- 1-pound shrimp, tails removed

Directions:

In a large skillet, melt the coconut oil over medium-high heat. Add the onion and cauliflower and cook until they are softened.

Add coconut milk, curry, and parsley to the skillet. (Feel free to add any other spices you like. Turmeric will give you an even bigger anti-inflammatory boost.) Cook for 2–3 more minutes.

Stir the shrimp into the skillet and cook until it is opaque.

Nutrition: Calories 332 kcal Total Fat 22g Carbs 11g Protein 24g Sodium 309 mg

27. Mango Chicken Meal

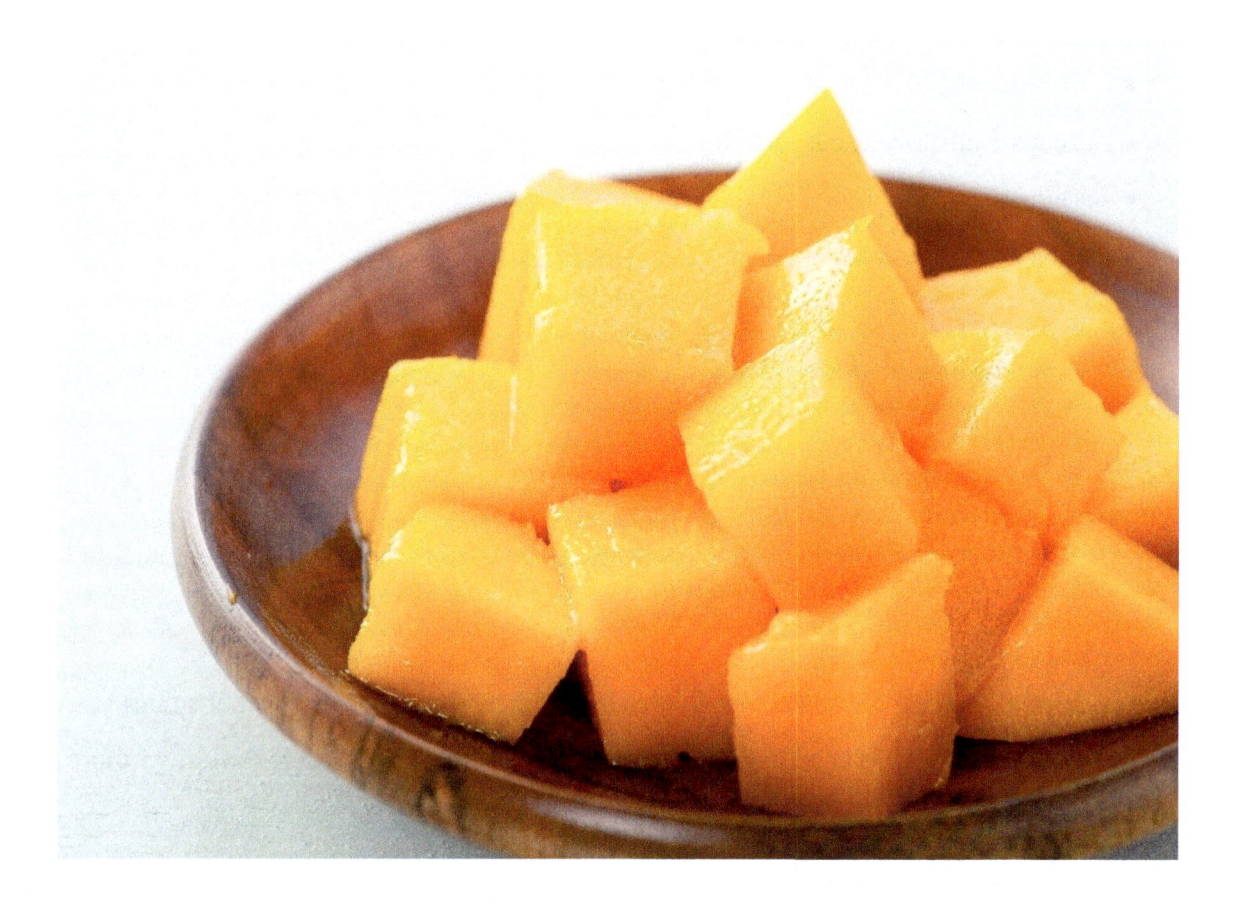

Mango Chicken is a popular dish in the United States and Thailand. The chicken is coated with a spicy, nutty, sweet sauce that coats the meat and creates a crispy shell on top.

Preparation Time: 25 minutes

Cooking Time: 10 minutes

Servings: 4

Ingredients:

- 2 medium mangoes, peeled and sliced
- 10 ounces coconut almond milk
- 4 tsp. of vegetable oil
- 4 tsp. of spicy curry paste
- 14 ounces chicken breast halves, skinless and boneless, cut into cubes
- 4 medium shallots
- 1 large English cucumber, sliced and seeded

Directions:

Slice half of the mangoes and add the halves to a bowl.

Add mangoes and coconut almond milk to a blender and blend until you have a smooth puree.

Keep the mixture on the side.

Take a large-sized pot and place it over medium heat, add oil and allow the oil to heat up.

Add curry paste and cook for 1 minute until you have a nice fragrance; add shallots and chicken to the pot and cook for 5 minutes.

Pour mango puree into the mix and allow it to heat up.

Serve the cooked chicken with mango puree and cucumbers.

Enjoy!

Nutrition: Calories: 398 Fat: 20g Carbohydrates: 32g Protein: 26g

28. Mediterranean Tuna-Spinach Salad

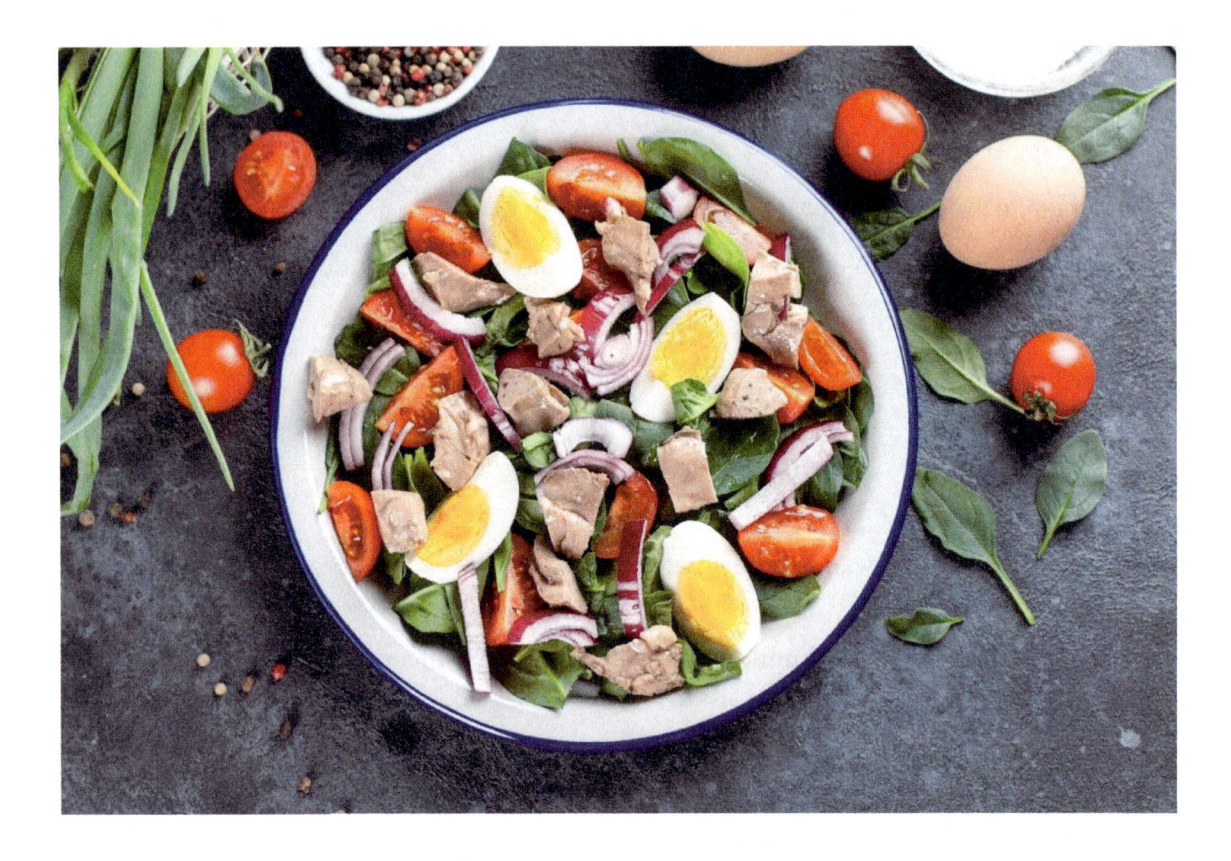

Mediterranean Tuna-Spinach Salad is a healthy, easy-to-make salad made with tuna and fresh spinach. This salad isn't the ordinary tuna salad that you have had before.

Preparation time: 10 minutes

Cooking time: 0 minutes

Servings: 4

Ingredients:

For the dressing:

- 6 tbsp. tahini
- 6 tbsp. water
- 6 tbsp. lemon juice

For the salad:

- 4 cans (5 ounces each) chunk light tuna in water, drained
- ½ cup feta cheese
- 8 cups baby spinach
- 16 kalamata olives, pitted, chopped
- ½ cup chopped parsley
- 4 medium oranges, peeled

Directions:

To make the dressing: Combine lemon juice, tahini, and water in a bowl. Whisk until smooth and well combined.

Stir in olives, tuna, parsley, and feta.

Divide spinach into four serving plates. Divide the salad among the plates and place it over the spinach and serve along with orange on each plate.

Nutrition: Calories – 376 Fat – 13.9 g Total Carbohydrate – 26.2 g Protein – 25.7 g

29. Lemony Mussels

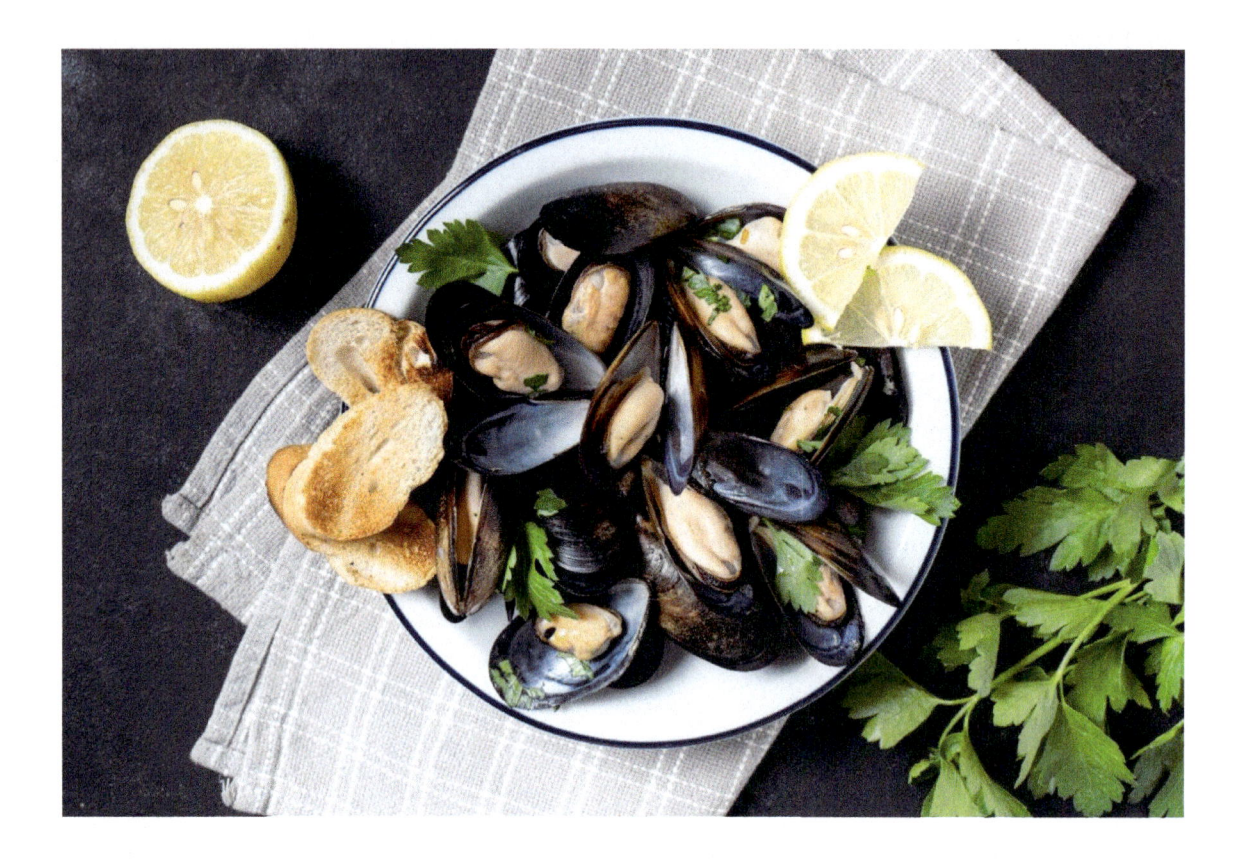

Lemony Mussels is a dish with ingredients including ground pepper, chopped lemongrass, salt, butter, garlic, and ginger. It can be served in several ways. Sometimes it is cooked in a lidded pan on the stovetop or in the oven; other times, it might be steamed or cooked over a flame.

Preparation Time: 5 minutes

Cooking Time: 5 minutes

Servings: 4

Ingredients:

- 1 tbsp. extra-virgin olive oil
- 2 minced garlic cloves
- 2 lbs. scrubbed mussels
- Juice of one lemon

Directions:

Put some water in a pot, add mussels, bring with a boil over medium heat, cook for 5 minutes, discard unopened mussels and transfer them with a bowl.

In another bowl, mix the oil with garlic and freshly squeezed lemon juice, whisk well, and add over the mussels, toss and serve. Enjoy!

Nutrition: Calories 140 kcal Total Fat 4g Carbs 8 g Protein 8 g Sugars 4g Sodium 600 mg

Snacks and Appetizer

30. Green Bean Snack

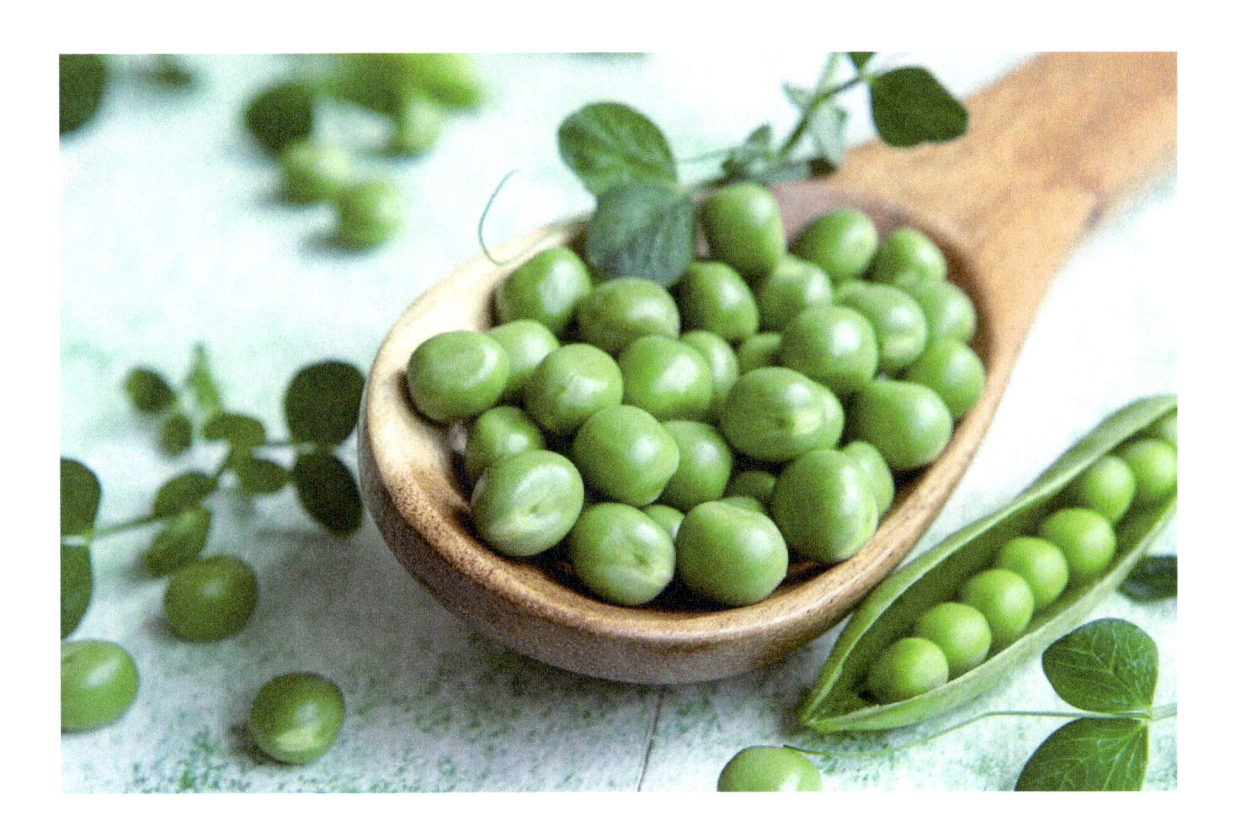

Green bean is a type of legume that is common in many parts of the world. It is made from green beans, salt, and water with other seasonings such as sugar, lemon juice, or vinegar.

Preparation time: 10 minutes

Cooking time: 8 hours

Servings: 8

Ingredients:

- 1/3 cup coconut oil, melted
- 5 pounds green beans
- Salt to the taste
- 1 tsp. garlic powder
- 1 tsp. onion powder

Directions:

In a bowl, mix green beans with coconut oil, salt, garlic, and onion powder. Put them in your dehydrator and dry them for 8 hours at 135 degrees. Serve cold as a snack.

Enjoy!

Nutrition: calories 100, fat 12, fiber 4, carbs 8, protein 5

31. Avocado and Pepper Hummus

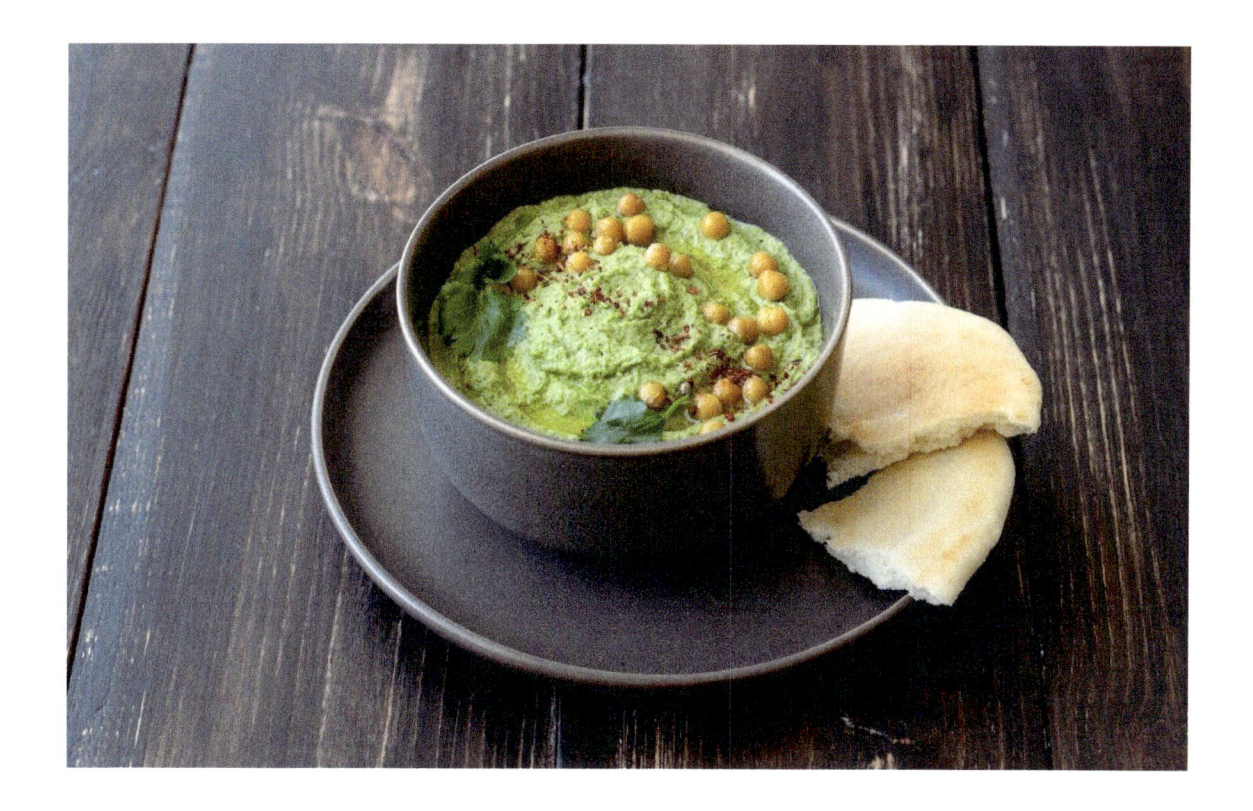

Avocado and Pepper Hummus is a creamy, spicy dip with a kick of heat. This flavorful hummus recipe is a tasty addition to any party spread or as part of your lunchtime sandwich.

Preparation time: 10 minutes

Cooking time: 0 minutes

Servings: 6

Ingredients:

- 2 avocados, peeled, pitted, chopped
- Salt and black pepper to the taste
- 1 tbsp. coconut oil
- 4 garlic cloves, chopped
- ½ cup tahini
- 2 tbsp. lemon juice
- 4 ounces roasted peppers, chopped

Directions:

In a blender, mix the avocados with salt, pepper, oil, garlic, tahini, lemon juice, and peppers. Pulse until smooth, then divide into bowls and serve as a snack.

Enjoy!

Nutrition: calories 140, fat 6, fiber 2, carbs 9, protein 8

32. Easy Eggplant Spread

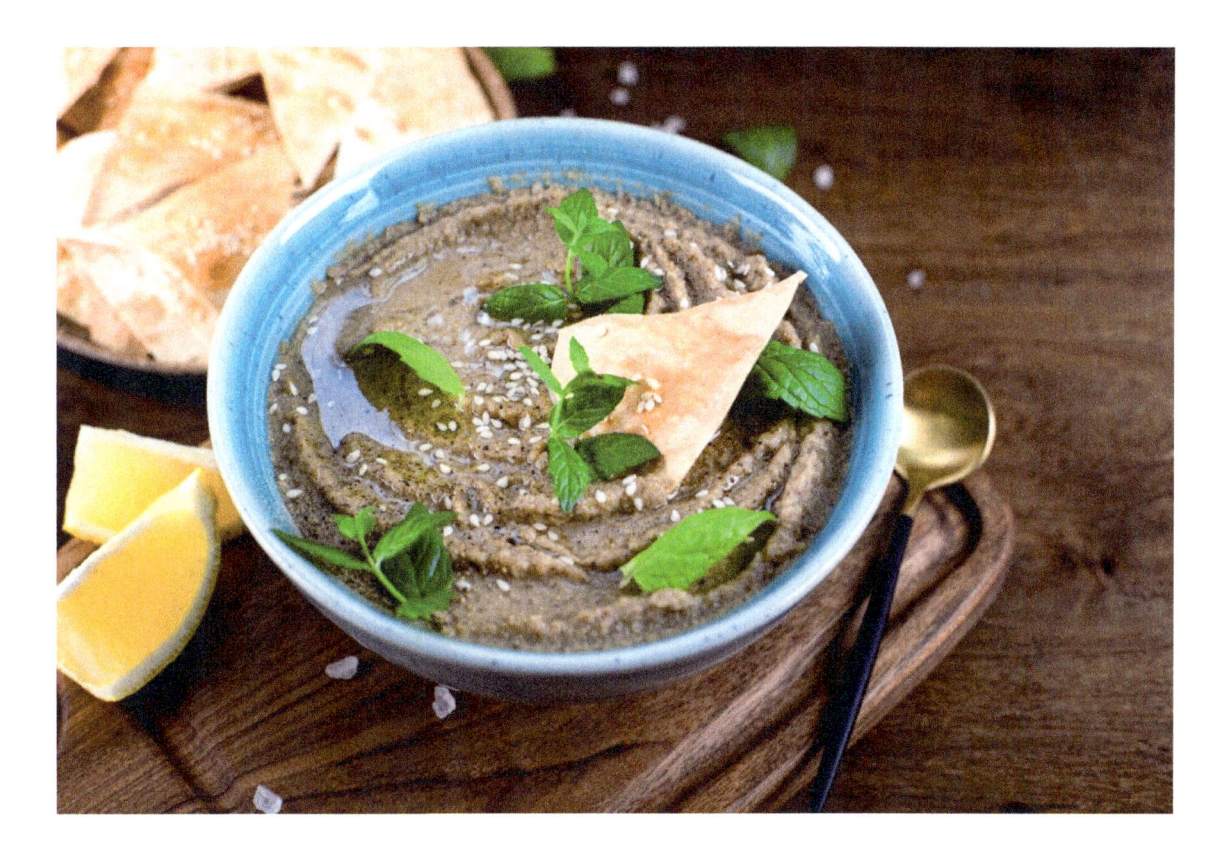

Easy Eggplant Spread Recipe is the perfect way to enjoy and share this delicious Mediterranean delight! This dish can be enjoyed on pita bread, oatmeal, or spread over a sandwich. It also has the added benefit of being vegan, gluten-free, and paleo.

Preparation time: 10 minutes

Cooking time: 0 minutes

Servings: 6

Ingredients:

- 2 pounds eggplant, baked, peeled and chopped
- A pinch of salt and black pepper
- 4 tbsp. olive oil
- 4 garlic cloves, chopped
- Juice of 1 lemon
- ¼ cup black olives, pitted
- 1 tbsp. sesame paste

Directions:

In a blender, mix the eggplant with salt, pepper, oil, garlic, lemon juice, olives, and sesame paste. Blend until smooth, then divide into bowls and serve.

Enjoy!

Nutrition: calories 165, fat 11, fiber 4, carbs 8, protein 5

33. Creamy Artichoke Spread

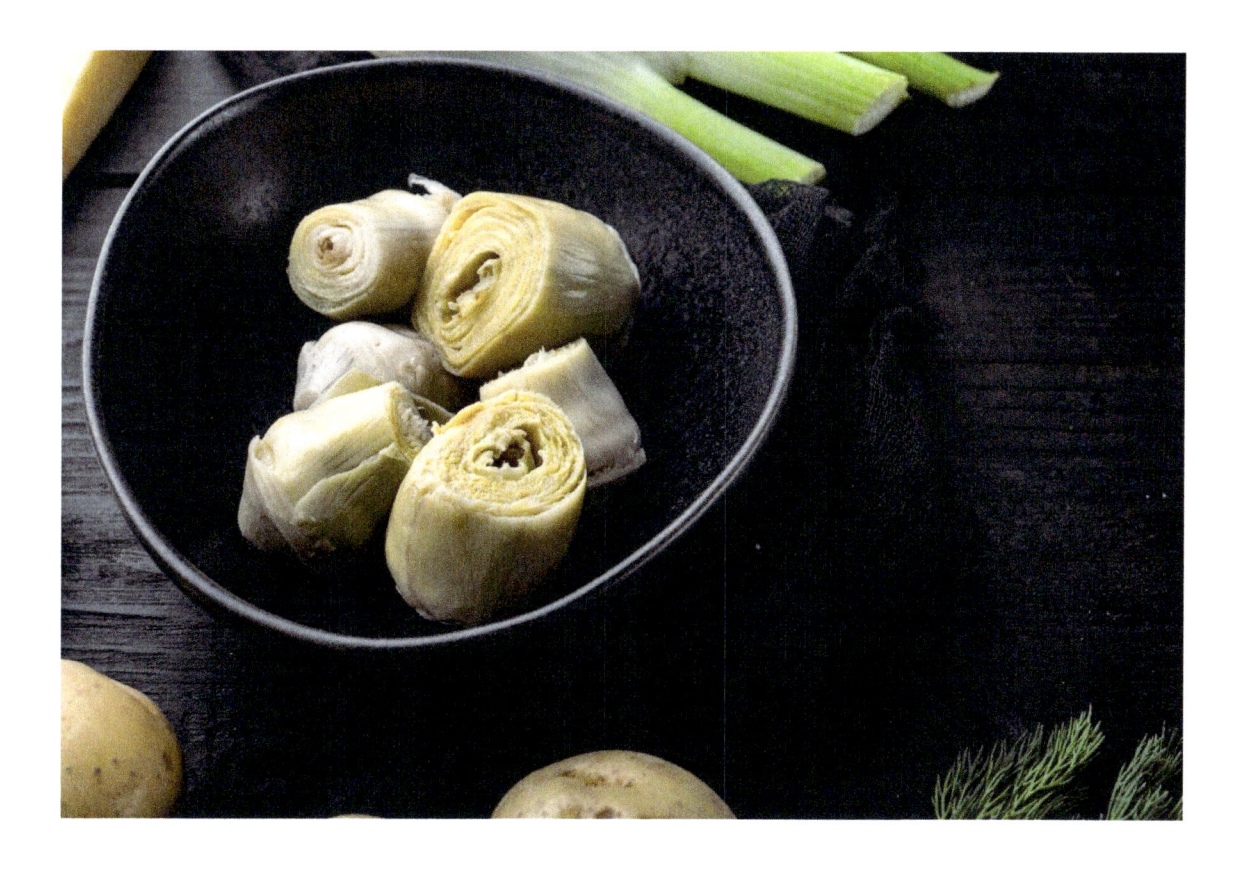

A creamy artichoke spread is a smooth, savory dip. It can be served with bread or crackers, as well as a variety of other dippers such as carrot sticks and celery sticks.

Preparation time: 10 minutes

Cooking time: 35 minutes

Servings: 6

Ingredients:

- 2 garlic cloves, minced
- Juice of ½ lemon
- 1 cup veggie stock
- 1 pound baby artichokes, trimmed and stems cut off
- 1 cup coconut cream
- A pinch of salt and black pepper

Directions:

In a small pot, mix the artichokes with the stock, salt, and pepper. Stir and bring to a simmer over medium heat.

Simmer for 35 minutes, then transfer to a blender, add the garlic, lemon juice, and cream, and pulse well. Divide into bowls and serve.

Enjoy!

Nutrition: calories 150, fat 2, fiber 3, carbs 8, protein 5

34. Balsamic Onion Snack

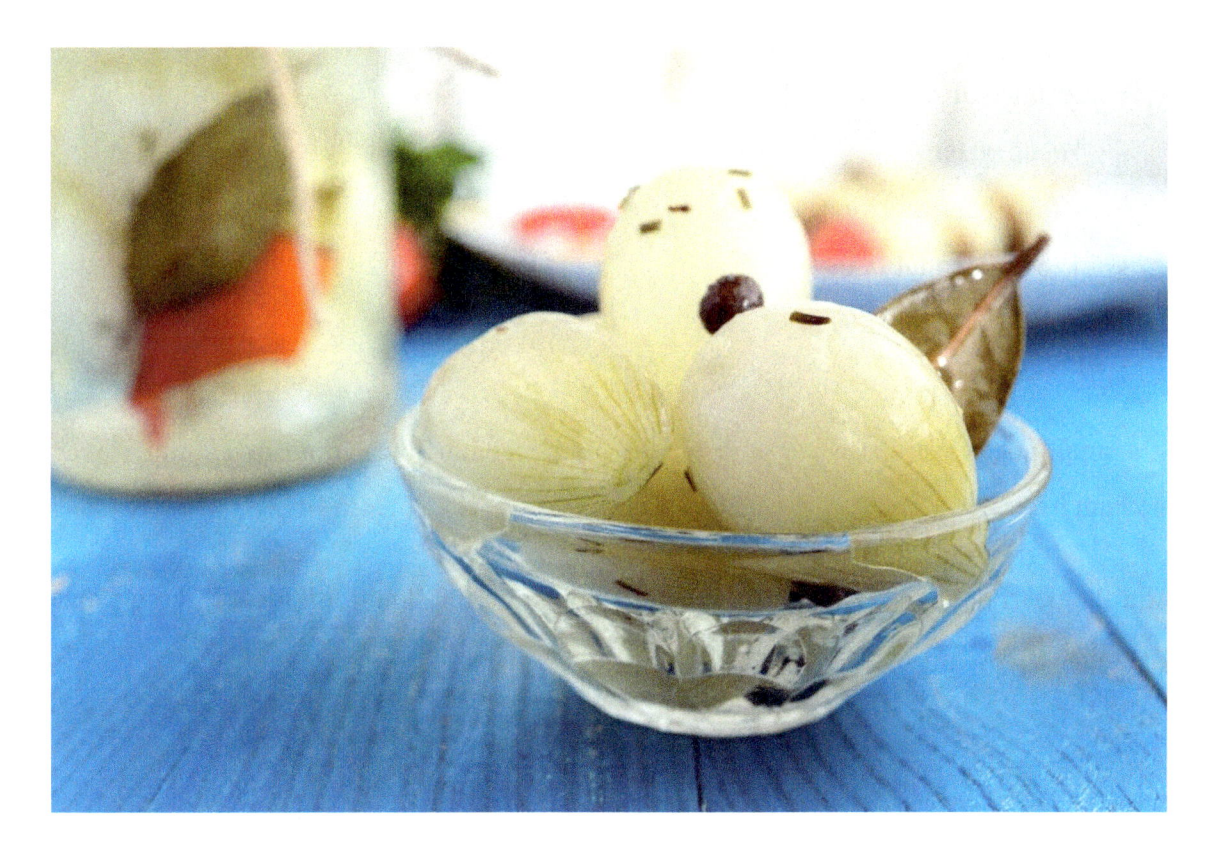

Balsamic onion snack is a great way to spruce up an uninspired lunch. It's also quite easy to make and can be thrown together in a matter of minutes.

Preparation time: 10 minutes

Cooking time: 10 minutes

Servings: 4

Ingredients:

- 1 pound pearl onions, peeled
- A pinch of salt and black pepper
- ½ cup water
- 4 tbsp. balsamic vinegar
- 1 tbsp. coconut flour

Directions:

In a small pot, whisk the water with vinegar and coconut flour. Bring to a simmer over medium heat.

Add the pearl onions, toss, cook for 10 minutes, drain the liquid, divide into bowls and serve as a snack.

Enjoy!

Nutrition: calories 100, fat 9, fiber 4, carbs 11, protein 6

35. Sweet Paprika Oysters

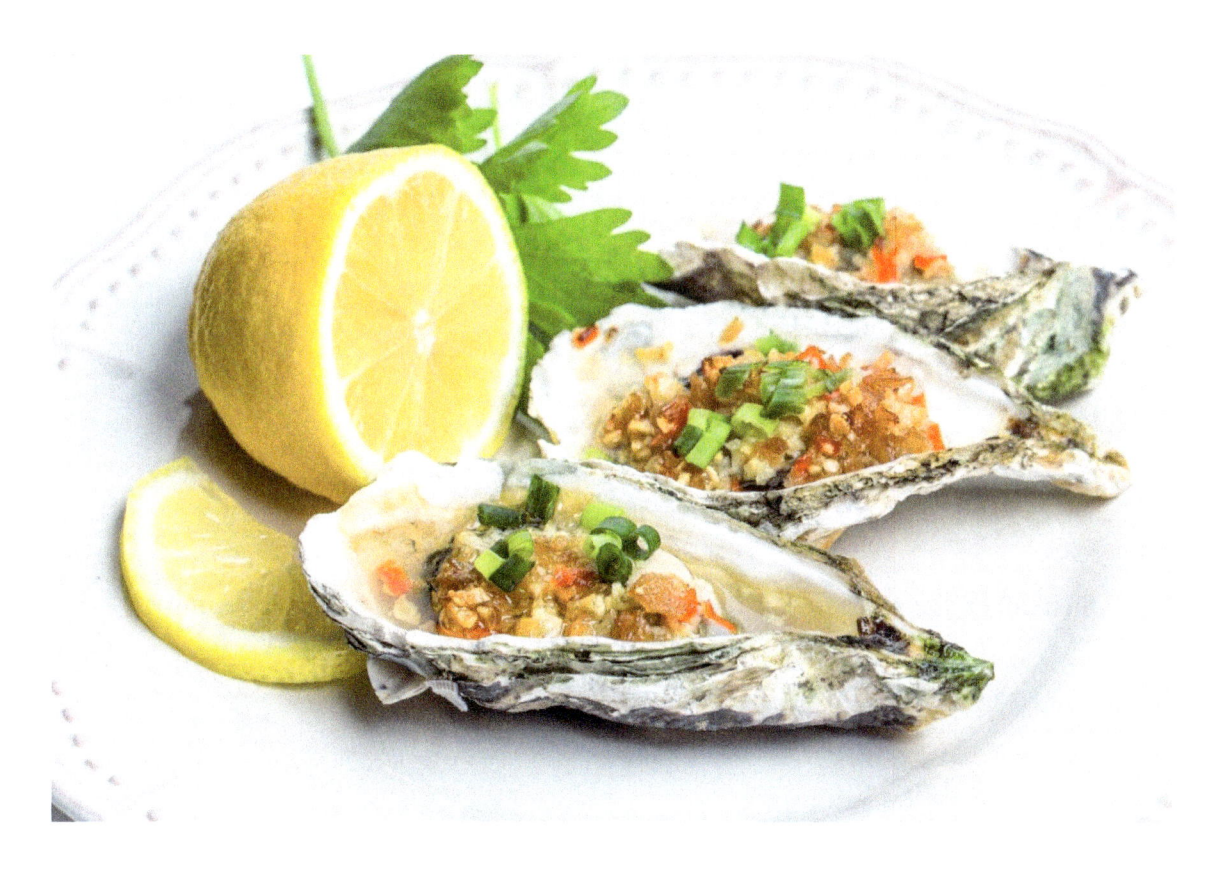

Sweet Paprika Oysters are a tasty and very easy appetizer that you can whip up in about 10 minutes. It's also one of those dishes where you can use whatever ingredients you want, so long as they are good quality and taste good together.

Preparation time: 10 minutes

Cooking time: 8 minutes

Servings: 3

Ingredients:

- 6 big oysters, shucked
- 3 garlic cloves, minced
- 1 lemon, cut into wedges
- 1 tbsp. parsley
- A pinch of sweet paprika
- 2 tbsp. coconut oil, melted

Directions:

Top each oyster with parsley and paprika, then drizzle with the oil.

Place them all on the preheated grill over medium-high heat and cook for 8 minutes.

Serve oysters as an appetizer with lemon wedges on the side.

Enjoy!

Nutrition: calories 127, fat 13, fiber 0, carbs 5, protein 4

36. Citrus Oyster Platter

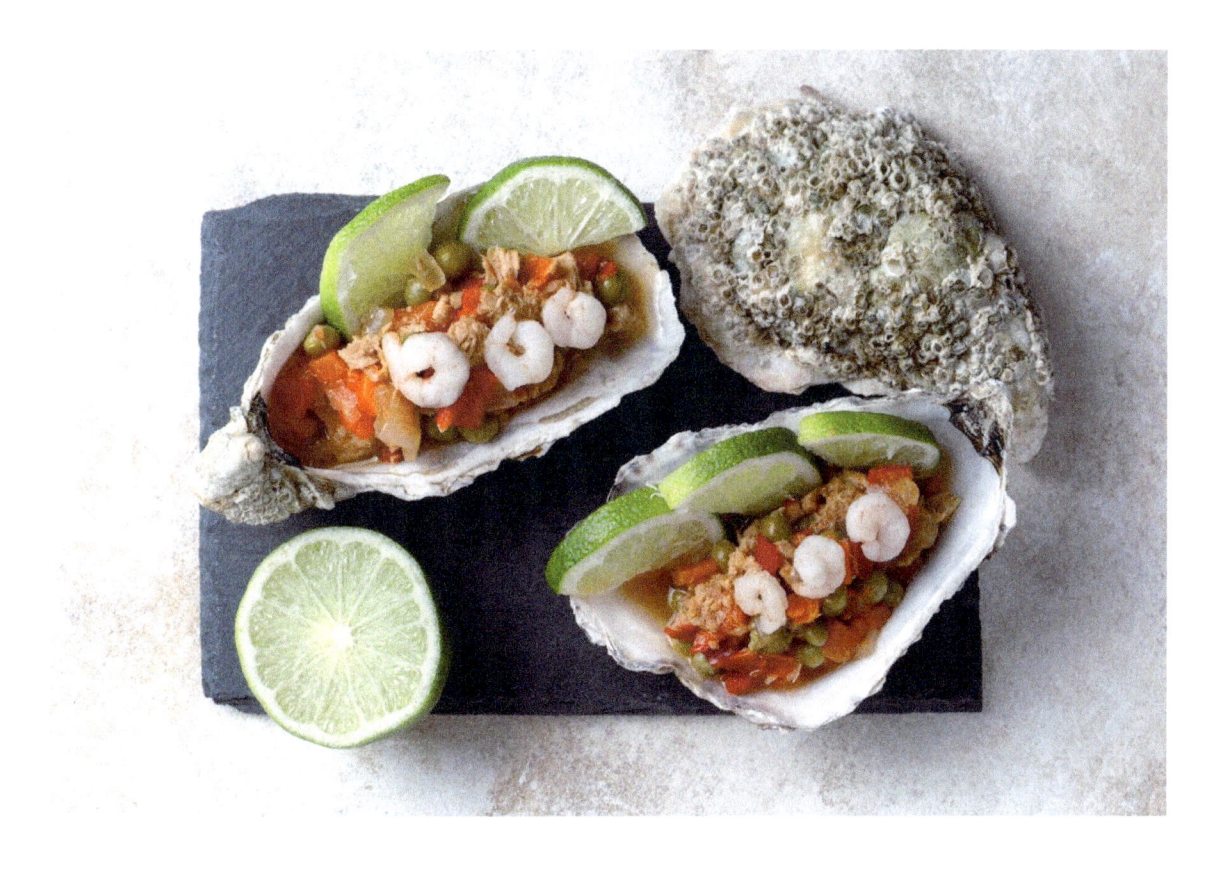

It is a beautiful and tasty dish that you can serve at any holiday meal or family gathering.

Preparation time: 10 minutes

Cooking time: 0 minutes

Servings: 4

Ingredients:

- 12 oysters, shucked
- Juice of 1 lemon
- Juice of 1 orange
- Zest of 1 orange
- Juice of 1 lime
- Zest of 1 lime
- 1 Serrano chili pepper, chopped
- 1 cup tomato juice
- ½ tsp. fresh grated ginger
- ¼ tsp. minced garlic
- A pinch of salt and black pepper
- ¼ cup olive oil
- ¼ cup chopped cilantro
- ¼ cup chopped scallions

Directions:

In a bowl, mix the lemon and the orange juice with lime zest, lime juice, orange zest, chili pepper, tomato juice, ginger, garlic, salt, pepper, oil, scallions, and cilantro.

Stir really well, then spoon this mixture into the oysters and serve them as an appetizer.

Enjoy!

Nutrition: calories 160, fat 8, fiber 6, carbs 16, protein 5

37. Salmon and Avocado Wraps

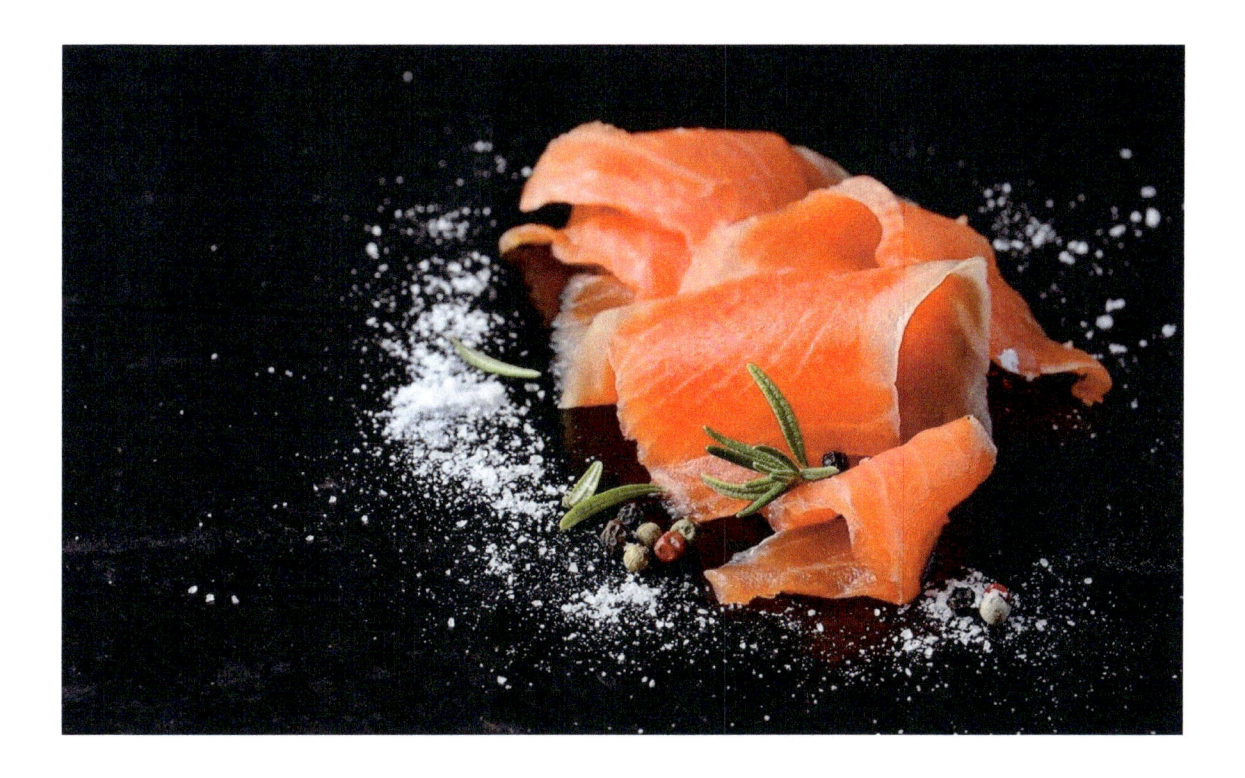

Salmon and Avocado Wraps recipe is made from smoked salmon, avocado, cucumber, fresh lime, and cilantro. It's an easy-to-make recipe with a great flavour combination of sour, sweet and bitter.

Preparation time: 10 minutes

Cooking time: 0 minutes

Servings: 12

Ingredients:

- 2 nori sheets
- 1 small avocado, pitted, peeled, and chopped
- 6 ounces smoked salmon, sliced
- 4 ounces coconut cream
- 1 cucumber, sliced
- 1 tsp. wasabi paste

Directions:

Place nori sheets on a sushi mat: Divide salmon slices, avocado, and cucumber slices on each piece of nori.

In a bowl, whisk together coconut cream with wasabi paste. Spread this over the cucumber and roll your nori sheets. Cut each into medium pieces and serve as an appetizer.

Enjoy!

Nutrition: calories 120, fat 6, fiber 6, carbs 12, protein 6

38. Radish Chips

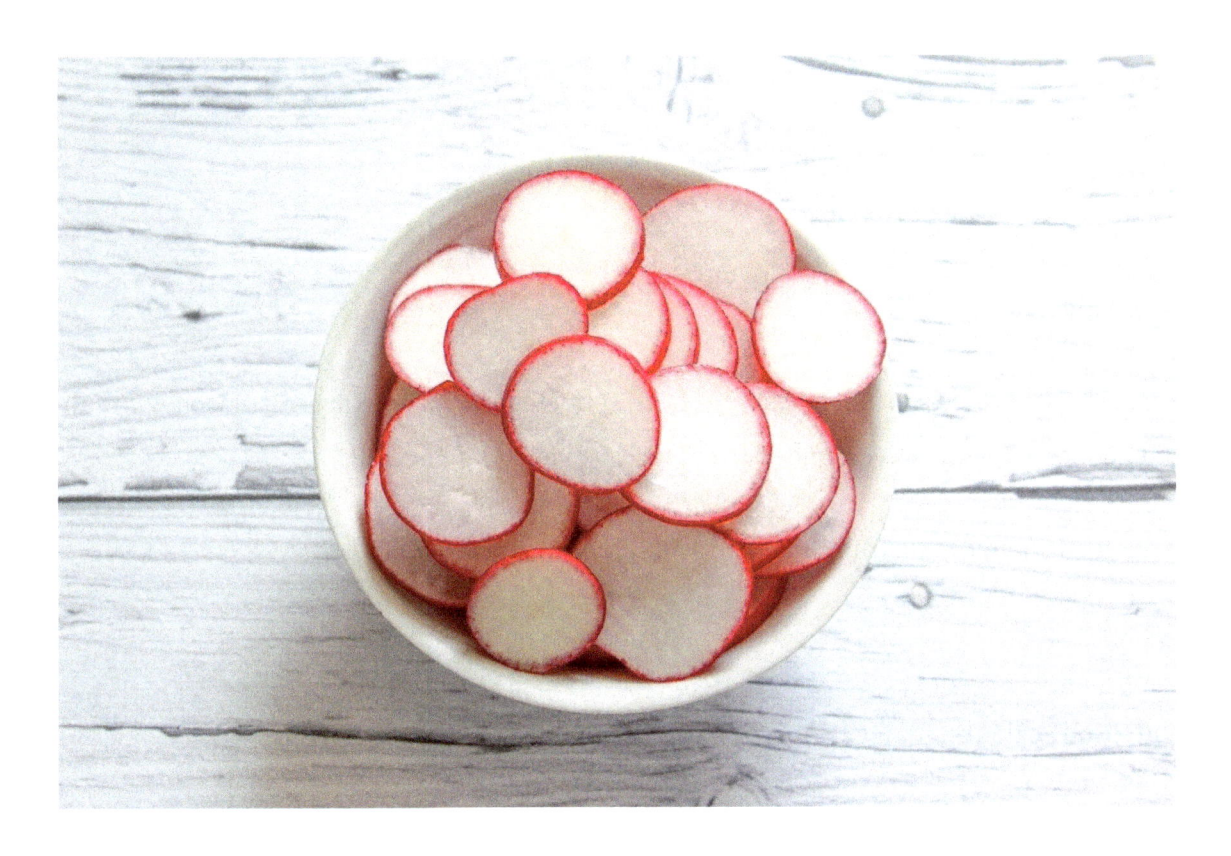

Radish Chips recipe is a great snack to serve at any get-together or party. It is also a way for you to enjoy the raw vegetable radishes without burning your fingers on hot strips of radish or having them turn into mush in your hands.

Preparation time: 10 minutes

Cooking time: 20 minutes

Servings: 4

Ingredients:

- Cooking spray
- 15 radishes, sliced
- Salt and black pepper to the taste
- 1 tbsp. chopped chives

Directions:

Arrange radish slices on a lined baking sheet, spray them with cooking oil, season with salt and pepper, sprinkle chives, and place in the oven at 375 degrees F.

Bake for 10 minutes on each side, divide into bowls and serve cold.

Enjoy!

Nutrition: calories 30, fat 1, fiber 2, carbs 7, protein 1

39. Avocado Cream

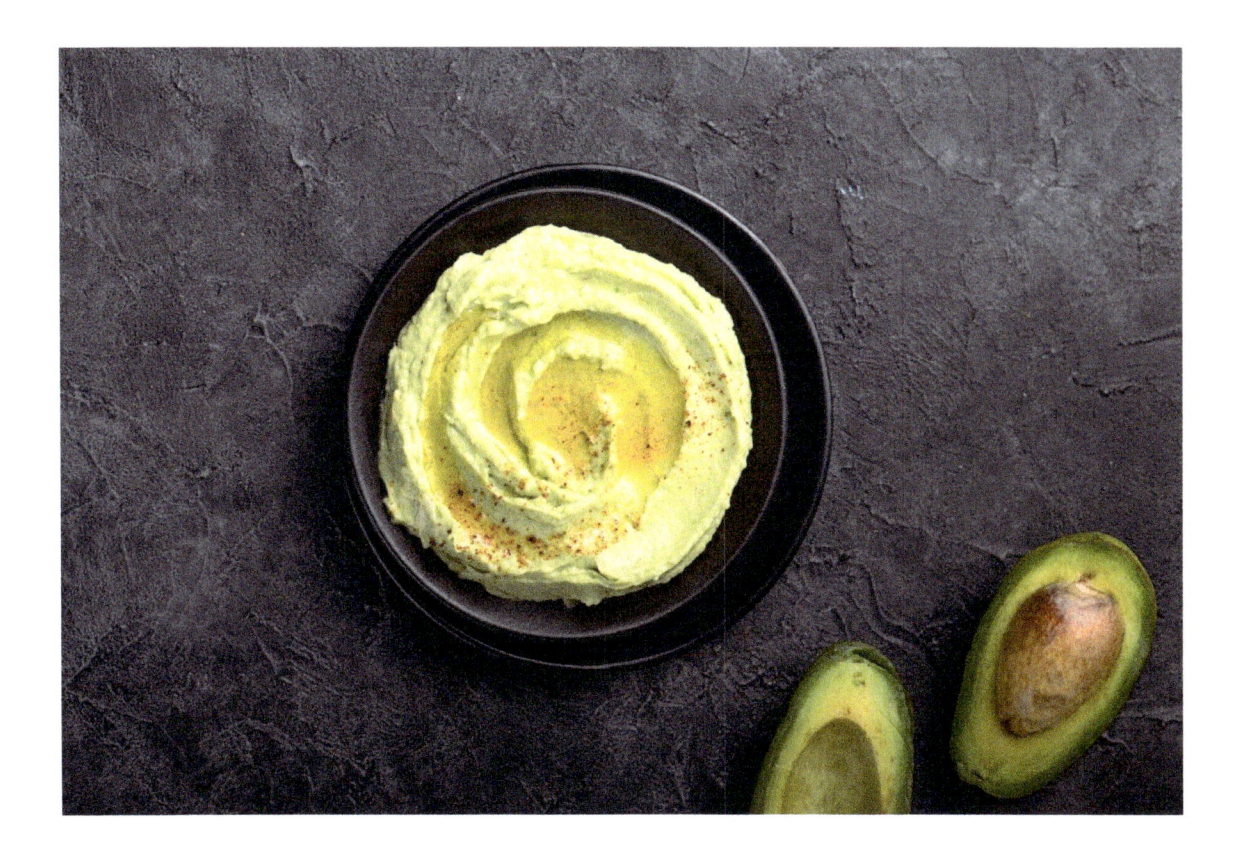

The avocado cream is a cold custard pudding with fruit and sugar that can be served either chilled or hot.

Preparation time: 10 minutes

Cooking time: 10 minutes

Servings: 4

Ingredients:

- 2 avocados, pitted, peeled, and chopped
- 3 cups chicken stock
- 2 scallions, chopped
- Salt and black pepper to the taste
- 2 tbsp. coconut oil
- 2/3 cup coconut cream, unsweetened

Directions:

Heat up a pot with the coconut oil over medium heat. Add scallions, stir and cook for 2 minutes. Add 2 ½ cups stock, stir and simmer for 3 minutes.

In your blender, mix avocados with the rest of the stock, salt, pepper, and cream.

Pulse well and add this to the pot as well. Stir everything, cook for 2 minutes, divide into bowls and serve cold as an appetizer.

Enjoy!

Nutrition: calories 162, fat 8, fiber 4, carbs 6, protein 6

Desserts

40. Orange Sorbet

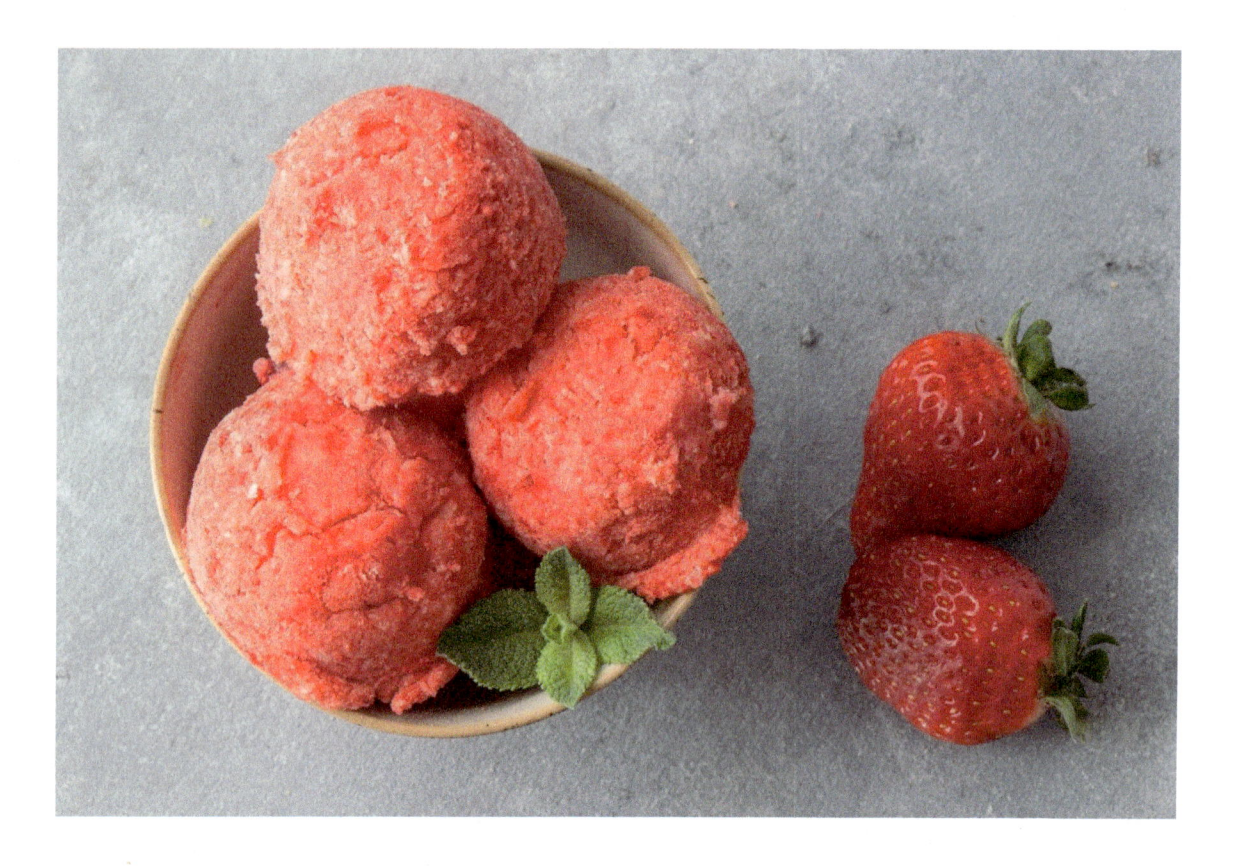

 Orange Sorbet is made with the juice of a few oranges, sugar, water, and naturally, lots of ice. It's not as sweet as ice cream due to the fact that there's no dairy in it. The sweet taste comes from just two ingredients orange juice and sugar.

Preparation time: 50 minutes

Cooking time: 0 minutes

Servings: 8

Ingredients:

- 1 pound strawberries, halved and frozen
- 1 cup orange juice

Directions:

In your food processor, mix the orange juice with the strawberries, pulse well then spread into a container. Keep in the freezer for 50 minutes, then scoop into cups and serve.

Enjoy!

Nutrition: calories 121, fat 1, fiber 2, carbs 9, protein 4

41. Lemon Cake with Pecans

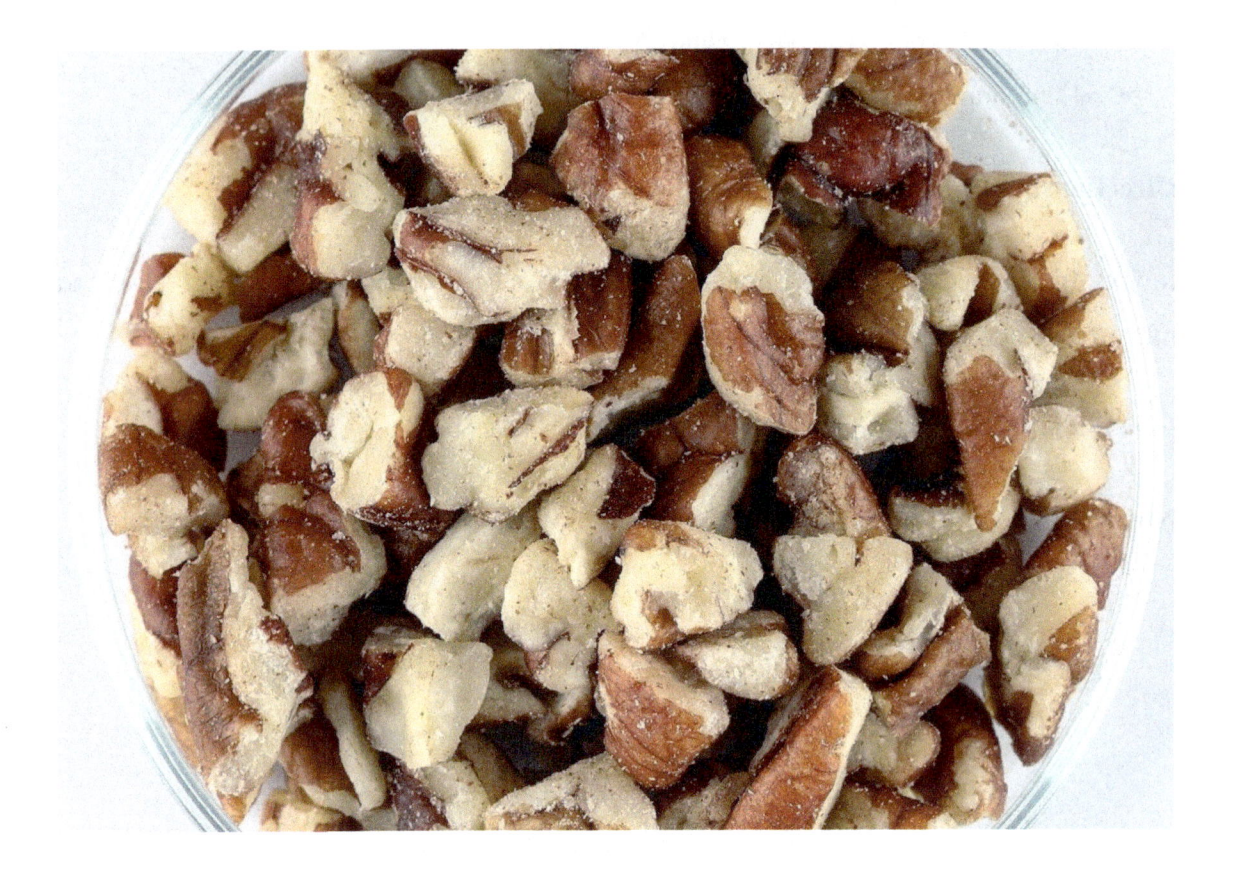

Lemons and oranges are used sparingly for their zesty flavor, but other than that, the dessert is not too sweet. The cake itself is light with a fluffy texture.

Preparation time: 5 hours and 10 minutes

Cooking time: 0 minutes

Servings: 10

Ingredients:

- 2 ½ cups chopped pecans
- 1 cup dates, pitted
- ¾ cup maple syrup + 2 tablespoons
- 3 cups cauliflower rice
- 1 ½ cups pineapple, crushed
- Zest of 1 lemon
- Juice of 1 lemon
- 3 avocados, pitted, peeled, and halved
- ½ tsp. lemon extract
- ½ tsp. vanilla extract
- A pinch of ground cinnamon

Directions:

In your food processor, mix the pecans with dates, 2 tablespoons maple syrup, cauliflower rice, pineapple, lemon juice, and lemon zest.

Pulse well, pour into a lined cake pan, and spread evenly. In your blender, mix ¾ cup maple syrup with avocados, lemon extract, vanilla, and cinnamon.

Pulse well, spread over the crust, and keep the cake in the fridge for 5 hours. Slice and serve.

Enjoy!

Nutrition: calories 215, fat 3, fiber 4, carbs 12, protein 8

42. Pineapple and Orange Smoothie

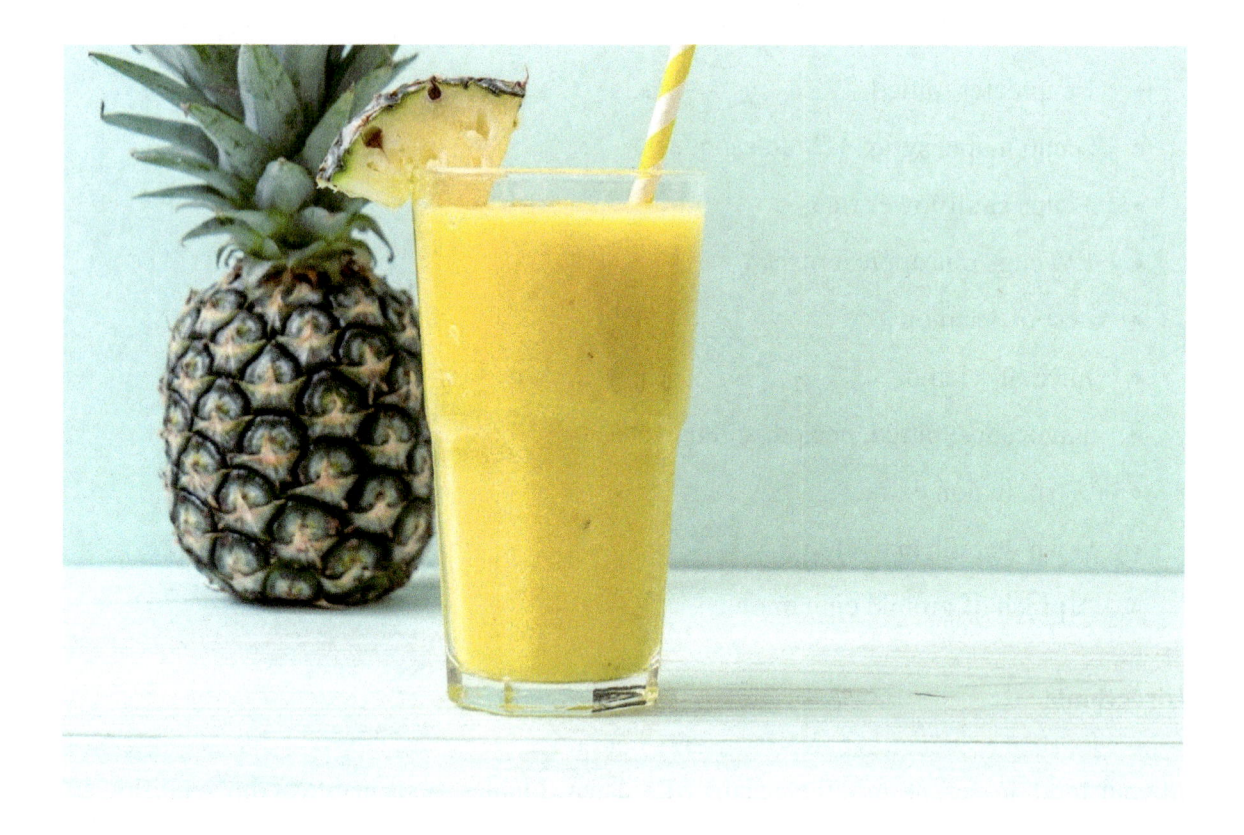

Pineapple and orange are the perfect combination for a refreshing smoothie. They go really well together in this recipe. Plus, pineapple contains bromelain, which helps to break down protein-based foods while helping digestion.

Preparation time: 10 minutes

Cooking time: 0 minutes

Servings: 2

Ingredients:

- 1 ½ cups pineapple chunks
- 1 cup coconut water
- 1 orange, peeled
- 1 tbsp. fresh grated ginger
- 1 tsp. chia seeds
- 1 tsp. ground turmeric

Directions:

In your blender, mix the pineapple with the water, orange, ginger, chia, and turmeric. Pulse well, transfer to a glass and serve.

Enjoy!

Nutrition: calories 180, fat 1, fiber 6, carbs 14, protein 3

43. Coconut Ice Cream

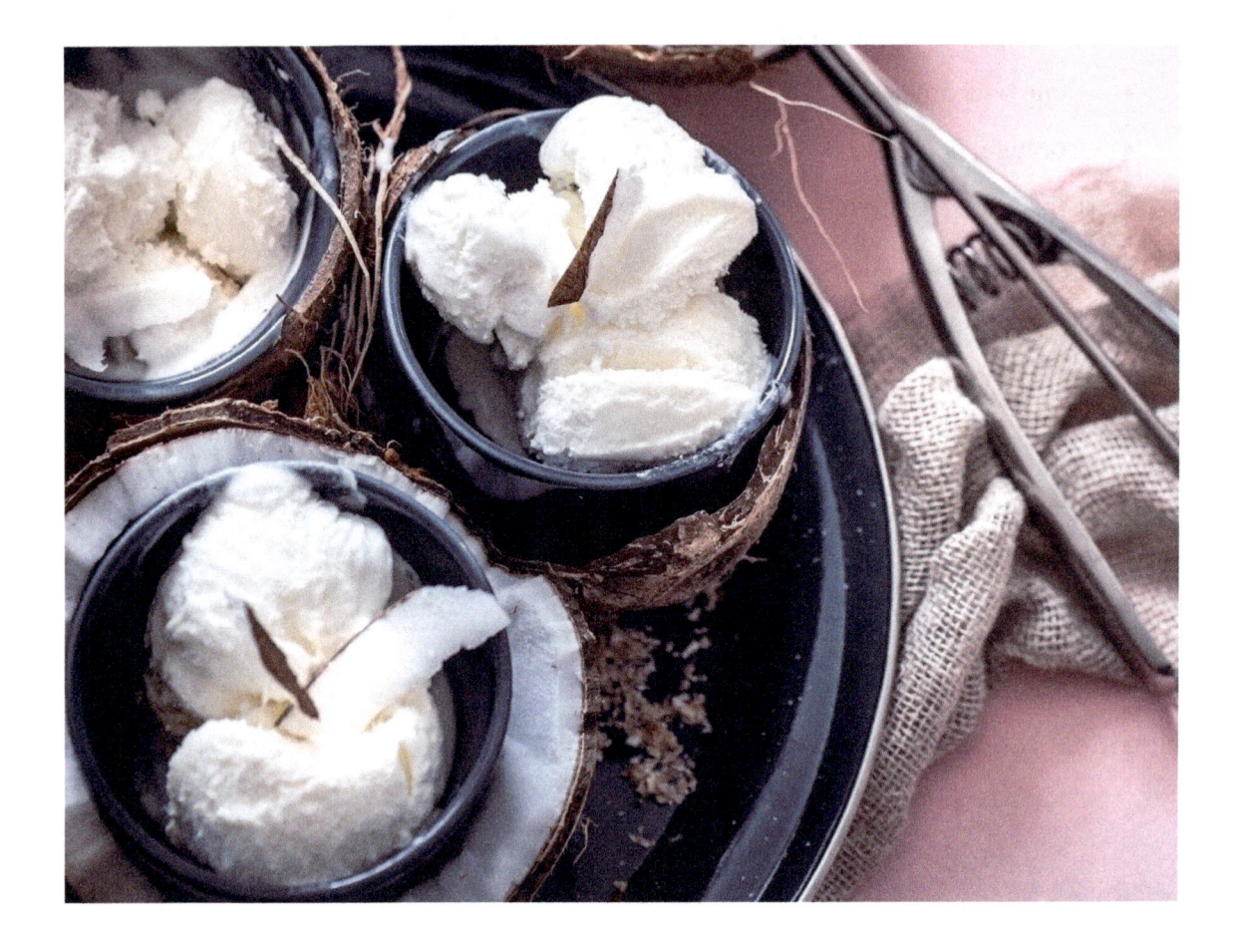

This is an easy-to-make dessert recipe that will satisfy your sweet tooth with the goodness of healthy ingredients like fresh coconut meat and full-fat canned coconut milk.

Preparation time: 8 hours

Cooking time: 2 minutes

Servings: 4

Ingredients:

- 28 ounces coconut milk
- 2 tbsp. fresh grated ginger
- ¼ cup maple syrup
- 2 tsp. ground turmeric
- ½ tsp. ground cinnamon
- 1 tsp. ground cardamom
- 1 tsp. vanilla extract

Directions:

Put the milk in a small pot, add ginger, maple syrup, turmeric, cinnamon, cardamom, and vanilla.

Stir, heat up over medium heat for 2 minutes, then transfer to a casserole dish.

Spread and keep in the fridge for 5 hours. Transfer the ice cream to an ice cream machine and process for 30 minutes, then freeze for another 3 hours before serving.

Enjoy!

Nutrition: calories 200, fat 3, fiber 9, carbs 12, protein 7

Conclusion

Thank you for making it to the end. The symptoms of ulcerative colitis can be caused by a number of factors, one being stress. Stress can contribute to ulcerative colitis by making your body produce excess amounts of substances that cause inflammation in the digestive system and irritate the intestines. Colon damage and malabsorption are common symptoms associated with ulcerative colitis, as is stomach pain.

Among the many health problems associated with ulcerative colitis, bowel inflammatory disease (also known as inflammatory bowel disease or IBD) is one of the most prominent. Bowel inflammation, mostly in the form of ulcerative colitis, is a disease that affects millions of people worldwide. This disease leads to inflammation in the intestines, which can cause watery diarrhea and abdominal pain. Bowel inflammatory disease occurs when the body's immune system attacks the thin lining of the intestines, causing blood loss and swelling in your digestive tract.

There are different kinds of bowel inflammatory diseases, including ulcerative colitis, Crohn's Disease, and regional enteritis. While they all have similar symptoms, they affect different regions of your digestive tract. Crohn's disease is an inflammation of your small intestine and colon, while regional enteritis affects the small intestine only. Ulcerative colitis is the most common kind of bowel disease among people in the developed world, affecting an estimated 600,000 Americans. The disease occurs when the body's immune system starts attacking healthy tissue in the intestines. This disease is common among women and people older than 50.

While ulcerative colitis can be treated with medication that helps control pain and symptoms, a diet where you eat foods proven to help heal ulcerative colitis is also an option. The most reliable way of curing ulcerative colitis is by changing your diet and eating foods that help improve intestinal health. Fruits and vegetables like cauliflower, carrots, and broccoli have been proven to be an effective treatment for ulcerative colitis.

I hope you liked this book!

About the Author

Since he was a child, Logan King enjoyed watching his mom cook. For him, it was even more fun than playing with his friends. That's how he fell in love with cooking. In fact, the first thing he ever cooked on his own was a cupcake, a surprise for his little sister, which not even his mom was expecting.

Now, supported by the whole family he is constantly sharing new recipes of his own creations. He finished a gastronomy academy when he was 18 and continued his career as a chef and recipe developer.

Now his goal is to educate and help people fell in love with cooking as he did. Actually, he is advising mothers and fathers to give their children an opportunity in the kitchen, because they never know, maybe their kid could be the next top chef.

Even though he pursued a career as a chef, his cookbooks are designed for everyone, with and without cooking experience. He even says, "even if you don't know where your knife is you will be able to do my recipes."

The gastronomy field is large and there is no end in the options, ingredient combinations, and cooking techniques. That's why he tries his best to keep his audience informed about the newest recipes, and even give them a chance to modify his recipes so that they can find a new one, one that they can call their own.

Appendices

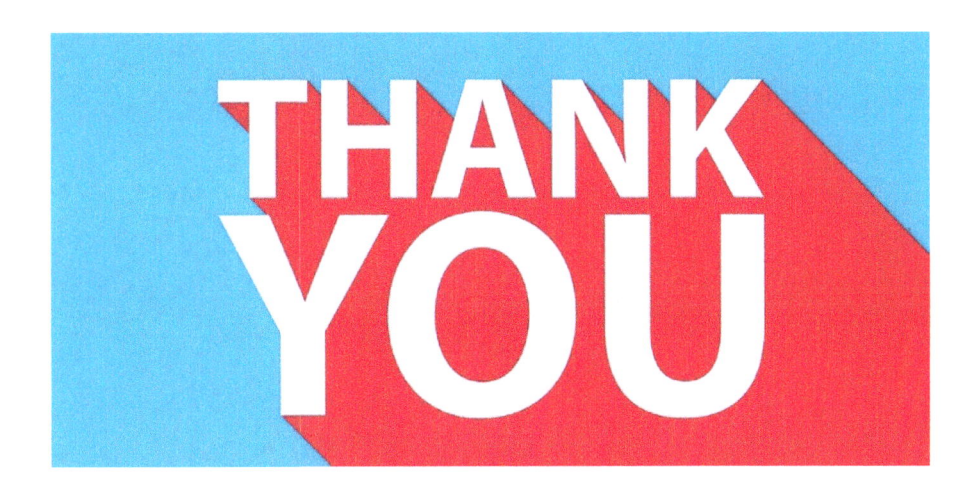

I am not stopping with this book. There are going to a lot more so make sure you are ready for the amazing recipes that you will be able to get from me. You can always be sure that they are going to be simple and easy to follow.

But thank you for choosing my book. I know that you haven't made a mistake and you will realize that too, well, as soon as you start making the recipes.

Please do share your experience about the written as well as the practical part of this book. Leave feedback that will help me and other people, I'll greatly apricate this.

Thank you once more

Have a great adventure with my book

Yours Truly

Logan King